MUSCLE POWER, MIND POWER

Building the Strength to Embrace the Beautiful Mess of Transformation, No Matter What the Scale Says

By:

LISA LABRE

The Pre-Game Huddle!

As you read what I promise will be an honest (and occasionally delightfully unhinged) exploration of muscle and mindset, don't be a stranger! I'd love to hear what lands with you.

Let's talk about building strength (both the bicep kind *and* the brain kind!), laugh over the absurd things we've all done in the name of health and fitness, and celebrate the wonderfully messy process of transformation together.

You can find me attempting feats of strength in these corners of the internet:

- **Website:** musclepowermindpower.com
- **Email:** musclepowermindpower@gmail.com
- **Instagram:** @li_labre

Dedication

To my brother, my mom, my boyfriend, and the
three personal trainers who, in their own unique ways,
have helped me build the strength, both inside and out,
to become the woman I am today.

To my little brother, Brent:

It was the long weekend in May in the late 90s, and Mother Nature decided to crank up the heat after what felt like an eternity of winter. The ice had barely melted off the lake back home, but my brother and I were itching to dive headfirst into summer.

When we were kids, my mom would take us to this private little beach with a boat launch. Feeling nostalgic, my brother and I revisited this childhood spot. The car was barely in park before we were both running onto the launch. Tentatively, I dipped a toe in. The water was frigid, a stark contrast to the unusually hot late spring air. Fearless as ever, Brent jumped in. His laughter trailed behind him as he swam to the nearby beach and called for me to follow.

With a mix of bravado and sheer stupidity, I jumped.

The shock was instant. My limbs seized, and my breath was trapped in my chest. I was an excellent swimmer, but the icy water short-circuited my instincts. I couldn't move, and for a terrifying split second, I considered the possibility that I might drown.

Out of nowhere, a strong hand plunged into the freezing water, grabbed my wrist, and yanked me out onto the launch. My brother had sprinted the short distance from the beach when he saw me struggling. Shivering and gasping for air, I still managed to hurl a few choice words his way that I wouldn't say in front of my grandmother.

Sure, he'd goaded me into that cold, dark water, but I'd taken the plunge of my own free will.

In the story I'm about to share, I plunged into some deep, dark holes of my own making. If I had stayed there, I could have gone off the rails more than a few times. Thankfully, I had someone by my side, encouraging me through the tough times and pushing me to want and expect more from myself.

Brent, thank you for being that firm hand. You've always been there to grasp my wrist and pull me back from the brink.

I love you.

To my mom, Donna:

My mom was the oldest of ten kids. Her mom knew how to whip up a feast for a small army on a shoestring budget, a skill my mom inherited despite having only two kids. Thanks to my grandmother's example, my mom never got into the processed food trend that swept through the 80s and 90s. There were no microwave dinners or pizza pockets in our house. Growing up, home smelled like a comforting casserole or a roast simmering in the slow cooker. Even with a full-time job, my mom always made sure my brother and I had freshly cooked, healthy meals ready for us to demolish.

Or leftovers. Ten kids' worth of leftovers.

She never quite figured out how to cook for a family of four.

Throughout my health and fitness journey, I was convinced my mom had it all wrong. Who gets healthy eating delicious, comforting casseroles, right? I misguidedly hopped on every trendy food bandwagon. Açai and kale smoothie bowl topped with flax, chia, and hemp seeds with a drizzle of macadamia nut butter, anyone? The problem wasn't the food. It was indisputably healthy. The problem was that I never felt truly satisfied.

On the other hand, my mom's home-cooked cabbage rolls and shepherd's pie are nourishing, satisfying meals that remind me of a happy childhood where regularly connecting over family dinners was a non-negotiable. Over time, I learned that I didn't need to abandon the recipes from my childhood that I love so much to be healthy and physically fit. Recipes like her chicken and dumplings have inspired meals I make for my family today, bringing that same comfort and joy to my family's table.

Mom, thank you for teaching me early on about the value of sharing a good meal with loved ones.

But that's just the start. I'm grateful for so much more than that.

Thank you for chauffeuring me all over town so I could play any sport my little heart desired, instilling a deep love for moving my body. Thank you for those late-night chats over a bottle of wine, where we dissected every twist and turn of my fitness journey. Thank you for being my travel buddy, shopping partner, confidante, and dearest friend.

I love you.

To my love, Serge:

My running joke about dating later in life is that it's like a high-stakes garage sale. Everything is sold "as-is" and it's definitely "pre-loved." Consequently, it almost certainly comes with its own fascinating collection of emotional baggage. The game is to find that one piece with incredible potential, the one whose "dings and dents" aren't just charming but somehow also complement your own. You'd better have a sharp eye and quick reflexes, though! If you don't immediately spot that diamond-in-the-slightly-dented-rough and recognize its worth *to you*, the next shopper with an eye for quality certainly will, and you'll be left kicking yourself for missing out.

Serge, you are my most amazing, perfectly complementary find. You're the garage sale deal of a lifetime, and I'm never letting go.

You have endless patience for my quirks and have supported my crazy ideas without batting an eye. Every day, I come home to a big hug, a warm smile, a tidy house, and laundry that somehow seems to fold itself. I couldn't do what I do without your love and support. Without question, you've always given me the time and space to chase my dreams, asking for nothing but my love (and maybe my cooking!) in return.

Thank you for sharing your family and their love with me. Thank you for your support and encouragement. Thank you for being my rock and my soft place to fall. Thank you for being my greatest love and devoted partner in life.

Most of all, thank you for all the years you spent playing hockey that gave you your fantastic butt.

I love you.

To my three personal trainers:

Trainer #1, you have a light and energy that's simply unmatched. At a time in my life when I barely had it in me to drag myself out of bed, you somehow turned "can't" into "can," one tiny step at a time, transforming this self-doubting couch potato into a slightly less self-doubting gym potato. That tiny miracle was *everything* to me, the clear signal I needed that this was just the beginning. Thank you for believing in me before I fully could.

Trainer #2, I was always so impressed by your wealth of health and fitness knowledge, and our chats between sets about everything from glute activation to the best 90s hip-hop were pure gold. But what truly set you apart was how you connected with people. The way you encouraged me, with just the right amount of cheesy enthusiasm, made me feel like I could do anything. You helped me redefine what was possible for my body and my health. That mindset shift led to a deep appreciation for the transformative power of strength training. For turning me into one of those crazy people who *loves* leg day, you'll always have a special place in my heart.

Trainer #3, when I first saw you in the gym, your intensity was undeniable. That "resting gym face" could melt steel. You were the master of tough love who wouldn't let his clients settle for anything less than their very best. But as I got to know you, I discovered your incredible empathy. It's a quality that gives you an intuitive sense of what your clients need and an understanding of how to encourage us in just the right way to strive for our potential. Your legendary workouts are equal parts brutal and exhilarating. Even though I curse your name and question my life choices mid-squat, I still jump out of bed and throw on my gym clothes the minute my alarm goes off, excited for our next session. You've taught me to dream bigger and set bolder goals for myself. To me, you're a brilliant coach, a valued mentor, and a ridiculously loveable goofball who also happens to be a trusted friend. I'm always all in for whatever crazy (and probably heavy!) challenge you have in store for us next.

To all three of you, thank you from the bottom of my heart for bringing your strengths and talents to my corner. You're miracle workers, life-changers, and the best hype squad a girl could ask for.

For that (and so much more!), I love all three of you, too.

Table of Contents

Introduction

I used to hate flying.

   As a person living in a larger body, it was always an ordeal. Filled with panic, I boarded the plane, dreading the look I knew I would get from my unfortunate seatmate. You know the look I'm talking about. It usually consists of a half-eye roll combined with a resigned expression when they realize their flight will be uncomfortable because I'll be spilling over my seat and encroaching on their personal space. I'd squeeze into my seat, anxiety spiking as I confronted the next hurdle, the dreaded seat belt. Would it even reach around my hips, or would I need to ask for the extender?

Although my first flight after my transformation started in the same way, things unfolded very differently. As I approached my row, my seatmate barely glanced in my direction. I stowed my bag in the overhead compartment, sat down, and reached for the seat belt. Without thinking, I loosened it to fit over my hips. To my disbelief, it didn't just fasten, but I had to tug it tighter. Much tighter.

It took a moment for it to sink in.

For the first time, I had room to spare in my seat. No more sitting at an awkward angle, hunching my shoulders to minimize my sprawl. No more desperately squeezing my thighs together, willing them to take up less space. After years of suffocating in a life too small, cramming myself into clothes and situations that never fit, I wasn't just fitting into the seat, I was fitting into my life. I felt like I could finally breathe and take up the space I deserved to occupy all along. Tears welled in my eyes, and I couldn't stop them from spilling over. A kind flight attendant noticed my silent sobs and offered a comforting hug when I explained the unexpected wave of emotion.

It's a moment I'll remember forever, and it became the catalyst for this book.

That moment on the airplane was a long time coming. My body and I used to be on good terms, but in my early adult years, we had a major falling out. It was a time of upheaval and uncertainty as I tried to find my place in the world. My weight steadily climbed as food became my go-to coping mechanism. By my late thirties, I weighed nearly 300 pounds. I felt lost, and the threat of a Type 2 diabetes diagnosis was a blaring alarm that my health was on a collision course with disaster.

I was a chronic dieter, forever chasing the elusive "perfect" body. From cabbage soup cleanses to low-carb crazes, I'd tried them all. Every diet promised a shortcut to happiness and self-acceptance, but they all boiled down to the same miserable mantra.

Restrict and sacrifice.

Back then, those words felt empowering, like I was taking charge and showing discipline. I believed I had to suffer to deserve the body I wanted. The more I restricted myself, the more obsessed I became with food. The more I sacrificed, the more I felt deprived. The harder I fought for control, the more I lost it.

My approach to exercise was equally misguided. I never moved my body for fun. It was always a punishment for overeating or a way to "earn" a future indulgence. My inner critic, who was about as kind as a ruthless queen bee straight out of a high school bullying nightmare, barked orders and made cruel deals like, "Burn 100 more calories, and you'll *earn* that glass of wine!" as I miserably slogged away on the elliptical. Exercise was never a celebration of what my body could do. It was a desperate attempt to fix what I thought was wrong with it. It didn't help that my inner critic was always there, ready with her unsolicited commentary, ensuring I never forgot how "unworthy" I was.

I felt trapped, losing the "restrict and sacrifice" battle on repeat. I knew there *had* to be a better way (that didn't involve *another* juice cleanse). Desperate for a different outcome and real answers, I sought help from medical professionals. You can imagine my deflation when I wasn't met with a fresh perspective or an innovative solution, but the same frustratingly standard cookie-cutter advice: "Eat less, move more." I knew they meant well, but that advice felt like my old "restrict and sacrifice" nemesis, cleverly disguised in a sensible lab coat.

If fat loss was as simple as "eat less, move more" or "restrict and sacrifice", this book could end here.

But after two decades of wrestling with obesity, I knew the reality was far more nuanced than that. Deep down, I understood the "restrict and sacrifice" approach was damaging, both physically and mentally. Labeling foods as "good" or "bad" fueled my unhealthy relationship with food, and using exercise as punishment sucked the joy out of movement and robbed me of its many benefits. It ignored the mental and emotional toll, the years of negative self-talk, and ingrained habits that kept me stuck.

So if the tired advice to "eat less, move more" and its evil twin, "restrict and sacrifice," aren't the answer, what is?

For me, it was *Muscle Power, Mind Power*.

I learned that lasting fat loss goes beyond diet and exercise. It requires you to embrace an approach that nourishes your body, mind, and soul. For me, this meant focusing on two key areas:

1. *Muscle Power*: Building physical strength and reclaiming a healthy relationship with food and my body.

2. *Mind Power:* Building mental strength by dismantling the self-sabotaging thoughts and beliefs that held me back, cultivating a positive mindset, embracing self-compassion, and believing in my potential.

It was a process of exploration and experimentation, dedicated to discovering how I could care for myself in a way that truly worked for me, one that fit seamlessly into my life and felt easy and sustainable. And to my surprise and delight, fat loss became the pleasant side effect of prioritizing feeling good and being happy.

Sounds wonderfully *simple*, doesn't it? Almost too *simple*. Because if you're anything like me, *simple* isn't your style. *Simple* usually means I'm about to detour into a period of intense overcomplication before I finally figure it out. *Simple* is the scenic route, the option that reveals itself to me only once I've exhausted every other ineffective alternative. I am, at my very core, a "learn the hard way, repeatedly" kind of girl. So for me, learning to listen to my body's wisdom was (unsurprisingly) anything but *simple*.

This book exists because I've personally navigated the path of overcomplication, enthusiastically diving headfirst into every pothole the health and fitness world has to offer along the way. By sharing my impressive collection of missteps and the hard-won successes they eventually led to, I hope to give you the insight you need to make your path considerably less bumpy than mine. For a more practical guide, you'll also find dedicated *"Muscle Power, Mind Power"* tips at the end of each chapter where I outline the costly lessons and impactful takeaways I wish someone had handed me when I first started.

While I hope that the end-of-chapter takeaways will be handy, please think of this book less as a rigid, "follow every single step *or else*" manual, and more as a story told by your best girlfriend. It's packed with anecdotes to make you laugh and some personal truths that I hope resonate with your unique experience. I warmly invite you to take from my story what feels true for your life and confidently leave the rest. My own path was so rewarding precisely because it was *mine*, and yours deserves that same personal discovery.

So, what does a story born from that kind of personal discovery look like?

Since my path was a real-life experiment filled with its own particular blend of ridiculousness, resilience, and revelation, what I'm about to share aims for something a little different than your typical before-and-after highlight reel of workouts completed and pounds lost. It's an honest, first-hand account of the often unglamorous but profoundly human work of transforming your relationship with your body and yourself.

Reliving my story wasn't always easy, but it's been worth it. By laying it all bare, I've found a surprising depth of healing for myself. And it's from this place of healing that I hope to connect in a meaningful way with anyone who's ever felt lost, discouraged, or, worst of all, alone.

If you've ever cried in a fitting room because nothing fits, walked away from a roller coaster ride because the safety harness wouldn't buckle, or gasped for air after climbing a single flight of stairs, I don't just sympathize with your struggle. I know its name. I've lived through the isolating shame and disappointment of those moments. Every. Single. One.

They defined me, and they shaped my story. But they don't anymore. And they don't have to define your story, either.

When I first stumbled onto this path, my only goal was to lose weight. That's it. No enlightened visions of self-actualization or becoming my "best self," just a straightforward "make the number on the scale go down, *please.*"

I never imagined it would turn into an expansive and often bewildering odyssey of self-discovery that gave me so much more than a smaller number on the scale ever could.

Through the unpredictable ups and downs, the sweat and the laughter, and the public gym meltdowns that made me want to fake my own death, I figured out how to own every raw, wonderful, messy piece of my story. In doing so, I uncovered a reserve of "take-no-prisoners" confidence and inner strength I hadn't realized was in me, giving me the courage to go after the life I wanted, not just the body I thought I needed.

Connection, owning our stories, and consciously building a life we love—that's the heart and soul of *Muscle Power, Mind Power*. It won't be pretty and it definitely won't be perfect, but I promise you, it will always be real.

Let's go.

Muscle Power, Mind Power Tip #1:
A Word on Body Positivity, Weight Neutrality, and Self-Love

Self-love. It sounds so warm and fuzzy, doesn't it? But to me, it sounded like a load of BS.

When I hated my body and desperately wanted to change, self-love felt like a reward I hadn't earned and a luxury I didn't deserve. I didn't know how to motivate myself in a positive way, with kindness or encouragement. Harsh self-criticism was my only tool. Every extra pound felt like a glaring billboard advertising my shortcomings to the world. My self-worth was so tangled up in the numbers on the scale that I started to believe something was fundamentally wrong with me. I believed I lacked willpower, discipline, and the ability to achieve my goals.

Self-hate can be a powerful motivator, at least in the short term. It kept me focused, pushed me past the point of exhaustion, and helped me white-knuckle my way through incredibly restrictive diets and endless hours of cardio. But it was also a brittle foundation. Hate inevitably turned into resentment, and that's when it all crumbled. I'd find myself binging on anything in sight, gaining back all the weight I had lost, and then some.

I lost and gained the same 20 lbs for decades, driven by that negative mindset.

You'd think the body positivity movement would have given me hope, but the call for radical self-acceptance sounded more like

8

an insult to me. How could I love a body that felt like a burden, an obstacle to the life I wanted? The pressure to love my body first, *before* I could start to change, felt like another impossible standard I'd never be able to meet.

It took time, patience, and a lot of self-reflection, but eventually, the weight of those old beliefs lifted. I realized I didn't have to choose between loving my body and wanting to change it. There is a beautiful symmetry to embracing self-acceptance while also striving for growth. I wanted to start this book by exploring body positivity, weight neutrality, and self-love because this mindset shift may have been the most difficult changes I made.

But if you're starting from a place of self-doubt or even self-hate like I did, I get it. It might seem like a bridge too far. Please trust me, the path is there. For me, it was a gradual unraveling, a slow and deliberate dismantling of deeply ingrained beliefs.

Body Positivity

- *Myth*: Body positivity means you have to love everything about your body all the time.

- *Healthier Perspective*: Body positivity is about accepting and appreciating your body for its unique capabilities and beauty. It allows you to acknowledge areas you'd like to improve while celebrating what you love.

I've lost a significant amount of weight, but "small" or "petite" aren't words I'd use to describe myself. I'm pretty confident I have better-than-average muscle-building genes, so I carry more muscle than the average woman. I have thick, powerful legs, broad shoulders, and a set of biceps that could give Popeye an inferiority complex.

Did I worry about my arms being bigger than the average woman's?

You bet. That worry practically had its own lease agreement in my head.

But I got over that deep-seated arm-anxiety once I decided that I'd much rather make jaws drop with my killer double bicep flex.

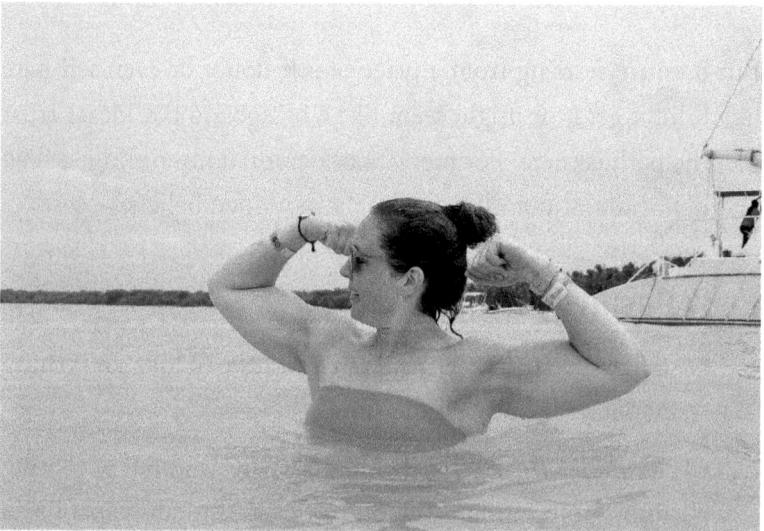

A tropical double bicep flex

Of course there are things I'd like to change about my body. Leaner legs and a bigger butt? Sign me up! But I've also learned to embrace my unique shape and appreciate my body's power and capability. In fact, that strength has ignited a fierce pride and confidence in my body, not just in how it looks but in what it can do. It's an unexpected advantage that allows me to crush challenges in the gym I never thought possible.

A few minutes on the fitness side of social media will show you that I'm not alone in this. A whole army of powerful women are challenging stereotypes as we crush it in the gym and in life. This is my brand of powerful beauty, and it's a hell of a lot more fun than chasing an impossible ideal.

Weight Neutrality

- *Myth*: Weight neutrality means ignoring the health benefits of weight loss.

- *Healthier Perspective:* Weight neutrality means prioritizing overall well-being and healthy behaviors, not chasing a number on the scale. If fat loss is a goal, it should be done sustainably and with self-compassion.

Initially, the scale was my best friend and worst enemy. I'd restrict calories and push my body to exhaustion, all for the fleeting high of seeing that number drop. My mood depended on it. If the number didn't go down (or worse, went up), my day was completely ruined.

My relentless pursuit of skinniness was a colossal mistake. In my quest to be small, I was unknowingly sacrificing muscle, the very thing that could have transformed my body. Losing weight without building (or at least maintaining) muscle makes you a smaller, slightly less squishy-looking version of your former self.

Everything changed when I shifted my focus from weight loss to getting strong.

Although muscle building is a slow process, I started seeing a different kind of progress right away. The scale's power faded as I celebrated victories it couldn't measure, like feeling stronger and more confident, having more energy, and sleeping better. Because muscle is denser than fat, my clothes fit better, even if the scale didn't budge. This disconnect between my weight and how I *felt* about my body led to a powerful revelation.

The scale was irrelevant.

I could be heavier *and* healthier, stronger *and* more confident than ever before.

Turning forty midway through my transformation brought a new awareness of the looming reality of perimenopause. Around the same time, a significant health scare hit someone very close to me. I'm a practical gal, so this double dose of reality spurred me to think seriously about the second half of my life. I realized how crucial muscle mass is for long-term health and independence. It's one of the few factors you can directly control when it comes to healthy aging and an investment in your long-term health and well-being.

With that knowledge, I now understand that I'm not just building muscle; I'm building my future. Getting older is inevitable, but surrendering to age-related decline is optional, and I'm not going down without a fight! I want to age powerfully and with vitality to continue living on my own terms. Muscle protects against a host of age-related issues, helps prevent disease, and allows you to maintain your independence. One of my most significant drivers for weightlifting today is that I never want to become a burden on my loved ones.

Weight training can give you a body built to last. And a body built to last?

That's *everything*.

Self-Love

- *Myth*: Self-love means never wanting to change. It means you're perfectly content with every aspect of yourself, and any desire to improve or grow means you're failing at self-acceptance.

- *Healthier Perspective*: Self-love means honoring yourself as you are right now while striving for your healthiest, happiest version. Your worth isn't tied to your goals, but self-love empowers you to reach them.

Self-love didn't come easy to me. It was far easier to punish myself with the familiar cycle of restrictive diets and endless cardio. My operating belief was simple. I would find self-love once I was "fixed."

And honestly, why wouldn't I think that?

Years of absorbing fat-shaming (both from others and, even more relentlessly, from myself), internalizing unhelpful medical advice, and battling the relentless societal pressure to be smaller had warped my self-perception. I was so ashamed of what I had done to my body that looking at myself in the mirror took an act of courage I rarely mustered. On the rare occasions when I did catch an accidental glimpse, the instant internal recoil was, "Ugh, look at you. You're an out-of-control mess." When you can't stand the sight of your own reflection, there's no way to grasp the idea that health and worthiness can exist at every size.

The thing about self-love is that it's a surprisingly natural process once you get out of its way. You can't force it with affirmations you don't believe or by pretending everything's fine when it's not. For me, it began to emerge when I ditched the fake-it-til-you-make-it false positivity and allowed myself to feel the full, messy spectrum of emotions—frustration, sadness, anger, disappointment—without automatically spiraling into self-hate.

The process was deeply uncomfortable, but absolutely necessary.

As I became more in tune with my emotions, I noticed these little moments, tiny glimmers of compassion or flickers of self-respect. However small, these moments became the building blocks of my self-worth, giving me hope even when I struggled with my body image. That's when I had a breakthrough. I realized that self-love is so much more than just a feeling. It's a *skill*. And like any skill worth having, it requires practice. Without action, it'll never grow. Without consistency, it'll never stay strong.

My journey with self-love has been far from perfect. There have been plenty of setbacks, bad days when old doubts crept back in, and times when I wanted to quit. But as I started to value myself more, I saw these stumbles not as proof of failure, but as a normal part of the process. Eventually, I saw them as opportunities to learn and grow. Each time I stumbled, I learned to pick myself up quicker, respond with more grace, and offer myself the compassion I'd previously reserved for others. What mattered most was that I kept showing up for myself, especially on the days when it felt like the hardest thing in the world.

There was a time when seeing my reflection felt unbearable. But I don't avoid the mirror anymore. Now, when I catch a glimpse, I find myself thinking: "*Damn*, that girl's a total badass!"

Weight Loss

- *Myth*: Weight loss is all about suffering and punishment. "Restrict and sacrifice" is the name of the game.

- *Healthier Perspective*: Done right, weight loss (or, more accurately, *fat loss*) is about self-care. It means fueling your body well, moving in ways you love, and prioritizing your well-being. It's not about deprivation, guilt, or feeling bad about yourself. When fat loss comes from a place of self-love and respect for your body, it becomes a sustainable and rewarding journey toward a healthier you.

You'll hear the term "weight loss" often, probably even from me sometimes, just because it's common shorthand. But let's make one thing clear. We're not chasing "weight loss" here. Anyone can lose "weight." You can donate a kidney, have a surprisingly productive bowel movement, or cut your hair, and voilà! Less "weight"! But unless you have the face shape for a pixie cut, that's not the kind of transformation we're looking for. What we're really after here is fat loss. And even more importantly, we're talking about doing that while we fiercely protect (or even build!) the beautiful muscle that gives your body structure and shape.

15

Back to the myth-busting!

The weight loss industry profits off your misery by selling crash diets and brutal workouts designed to make you hate yourself enough to buy in. I've fallen for that more times than I can count. "Restrict and sacrifice" burned me out instead of building me up.

My breakthrough was realizing that exercise shouldn't feel like punishment. Finding movement I enjoyed was the key. Lifting weights and cycling became a celebration of what my body could do. That kind of joyful movement made me want to eat well because I felt amazing and performed better. I knew the changes I was making would last a lifetime when fat loss became the welcomed side effect instead of the focus.

Maybe you look in the mirror and wish you could feel good about what you see. Maybe you're sick of fighting your body, tired of tearing yourself down. Maybe you're ready to build yourself up instead. In the following chapters, I'll share how I created a happier, stronger version of myself, inside and out, by ditching the "less is more" mentality and embracing "more is more."

More strength. *More* energy. *More* unstoppable confidence.

Muscle Power, Mind Power Tip #2:
A Word on Eating Disorders

Sharing my struggle with Binge Eating Disorder (BED) wasn't
an easy decision.

Eating disorders are incredibly complex and painful, and they can
have devastating effects if not addressed. It's vital to understand
that what helped me might not help you, and my journey is just
one among many.

If you're struggling, seeking help through avenues such as therapy,
counseling, support groups, or a registered dietitian is a sign of
incredible strength. There's no shame in needing support; it's
often the bravest step toward healing. There are people out there
who understand and will fight alongside you, as well as helpful
resources that will guide you.

Eating disorders thrive on secrecy, wrapped up tight in layers
of stigma and shame, and they do *not* discriminate. They affect
people of all experiences, identities, and walks of life. By being
open about my experience, I hope to show anyone who might be
fighting this battle in silence that:

- *You're not alone.* Stories can chip away at the isolation.
  Knowing there are others out there who understand can
  give you hope when you need it most.

- *There's no one "right" way to heal, and it doesn't need to
  happen on some arbitrary timeline.* While some folks
  experience spontaneous recovery from eating disorders

(and if you're struggling, I sincerely hope that's how it unfolds for you!), my journey has been more "long and meandering" than "direct and linear." As I'll prove over and over again in this book, learning things the hard way is my specialty.

- *Recovery is a verb, not a noun.* It's hard work, and an active, ongoing process. Some days, it might feel like you're taking two steps forward and one step back, but at least it's still movement in the right direction. While I've made significant progress, I don't consider myself fully "recovered." I believe healing my relationship with food and my body is a lifelong commitment to self-discovery and learning. I remain vigilant about the thoughts and feelings that trigger my unhealthy patterns. Even today, I still use the tools I'll share with you.

But I also understand that this topic can be deeply triggering. If reading about eating disorders feels unsafe for you, please feel free to skip Chapter 2 entirely. It's the only chapter where I go into the specifics of my battle with BED. Take care of yourself first, and I'll be waiting for you in Chapter 3 when you're ready.

There's still plenty here for you, I promise!

CHAPTER 1

The Graduation Dress

It was spring 1999, and my high school graduation was just around the corner. My heart was filled with a mix of excitement and that anxious feeling you get when you know things are about to change. In that moment of anticipation, I decided to try on the spectacular graduation gown my mom had lovingly bought me a few months earlier.

I removed it from my closet and carefully opened the protective garment bag. The dress was a vision in crimson satin with an elegant silhouette. The luxurious fabric cascaded to the floor, shimmering with tiny, dancing sparkles. It was the kind of dress that promised to make any moment unforgettable. I imagined myself dancing the night away as I stepped confidently into the next chapter of my life.

Princess mode, engaged!

But what happened next was anything but enchanting. As I struggled with the zipper, I realized the dress was more than just a little snug. It was a hold-your-breath, zero-possibility-of-eating-or-drinking-anything, stand-not-sit-all-night kind of tight. The disappointment felt overwhelming as tears welled up in my eyes, blurring my image in the mirror.

To truly grasp the weight of what I was feeling, we need to rewind. This moment wasn't simply about a dress. Years of feeling different because of my size had condensed into that one agonizing moment. It was a brutal intersection where my past and future collided. This moment was about a body that had always been strong, but also bigger than most.

I was a powerhouse growing up. I was taller, stronger, and more athletic than most girls my age. My parents selflessly sacrificed, scrimped, and saved so my brother and I could play any sport we wanted. We took dance and swimming lessons and learned the art of karate and kickboxing. We also played organized sports, like ice sports in the wintertime and baseball or soccer in the summer. On top of that, I played every school sport I could, including volleyball, basketball, and track and field events like running long jump, shot put and javelin.

The point is, I was always on the go.

There's one memory from when I was nine or ten that always makes me smile. The final school bell had rung. Instead of catching my usual bus home, I eagerly made my way to a different stop, the one for the bus that took me near my dance studio. With an apple from my lunch bag in hand, I walked the rest of the way, gearing up for a demanding two and a half hours of dance class.

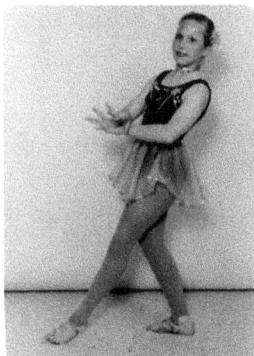

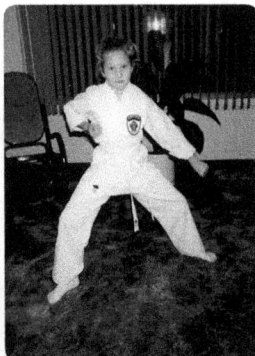

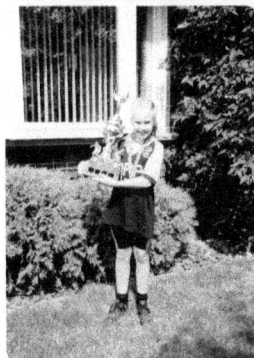

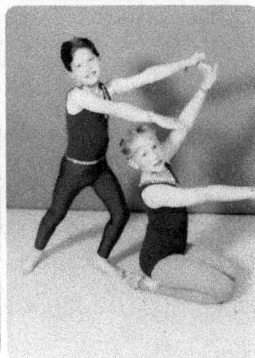

*I was a healthy, confident kid,
happily participating in any activity I could!*

After my final plié, I hurriedly packed my dance gear and school bag. I had to hustle because I knew my mom was impatiently waiting in the parking lot, probably checking her watch every few seconds. As I got to the car, the back door popped open. I jumped in, and we were off. Spread across the seat were my ringette gear and a sandwich.

With my mom weaving through traffic, I knew I had less than fifteen minutes to scarf down that sandwich and transform from a dancer into a ringette player. We pulled up to the arena, and she

21

helped me get my skates on. I hit the ice just in time for warm-ups and an hour-long game.

Hectic? *Absolutely.* But that was a typical Tuesday for me.

But before we go any further, let's clear a few things up.

What's ringette? Think hockey with straight sticks and a rubber ring instead of a puck. Back in the 80s, Canadian girls played ringette, not hockey!

You might also wonder about a kid taking herself to her after-school activities or not being buckled up in the car. It was the 80s! I was your textbook first-generation latchkey kid with two parents working outside the household. I had to grow up quickly, and I got used to being responsible for myself and my younger brother at a young age. So, finding my own way to dance class? No big deal. And back then, not wearing a seatbelt wasn't just expected, it was practically a rite of passage.

So, please, don't cancel my mom.

Back to the story!

Schoolyard dynamics can be harsh, and weight, unfortunately, is an easy target for thoughtless teasing. I got the odd comment hurled my way about my size, but they never really got to me. Thankfully, sports and my folks shielded me from that. Being an athlete gave me a solid sense of self and comfort in my own skin, and I inherited my mom's take-no-shit-from-anyone attitude and my dad's quick wit. Any teasing was quickly shut down, usually with a well-placed comment about my athleticism.

"You think I'm *large*? I sure am. A *large* threat on the ice!" Adding over my shoulder, as I walked away, "You know you couldn't beat me at the blue line on your best day, bud. Even if you had Gretzky's skates, you'd still look like a bag of pucks on the rink!"

(That's a solid burn for any Canadian who loves ice sports. If that isn't you, you'll have to trust me on this one!)

Even with all that confidence, I couldn't help but notice I was different. My friends were slender and petite, while I was big and sturdy. I felt a bit like a linebacker at a ballet recital, and I mean that in the best way possible. I saw myself as strong and capable, but I also understood that I wasn't the most delicate figure in the room. By some miracle, I managed to hold my own, even as the "heroin chic" 90s trend pushed many of my friends toward a rail-thin ideal.

Then came that spring day and the traitorous dress zipper. The societal pressure to conform was always there, simmering beneath the surface. That day, it erupted, triggered by a dress that suddenly felt too small and my youthful, carefree confidence in my appearance disintegrated.

Dieting wasn't just a thought anymore; it was the only way out.

Everything was different after that.

Graduation day was a bright red circle on my calendar, and I was desperate to feel beautiful as I celebrated this milestone with my friends. With my confidence rattled and the pressure of a looming deadline, my main source of information wasn't the internet (it was 1999, so the internet was still a clunky, dial-up mystery), but the glossy pages of fashion magazines. Up until then, I had been blissfully ignorant of diet culture. But those magazines? It was a full-blown indoctrination. I was instantly sucked into the world of impossibly thin models, miracle quick-fix diets, and the message that smaller was always better.

The damaging ideals of the 1990s and early 2000s left a lasting legacy on my generation of women. Many of us are still struggling to overcome the toxic messages we internalized during that era.

That's when I started my first crash diet.

Breakfast and lunch became an exercise in deprivation, a battle against the constant hunger pangs I desperately tried to ignore. Family dinners should have been a time for connection and shared nourishment, but they became my most elaborate and stressful performance. Any genuine pleasure in the food or the company was eclipsed by my hyper-focus on the charade. I pushed food around my plate to create the illusion of eating and took the tiniest bites to fool watchful eyes, while anxiously awaiting the moment I could discreetly ditch the evidence.

But even that wasn't enough.

I wanted to burn more calories, so I added secret workouts. I walked instead of taking the bus to and from school. I snuck in exercise videos from my mom's collection when the house was empty. When my family was around, I retreated to the privacy of my bedroom for heart-pounding sets of crunches and jumping jacks. The secrecy only added to the shame and urgency.

In retrospect, my approach wasn't just unbalanced and unsustainable. It was dangerous. But in that moment, it felt like my only option.

Fast forward to graduation night.

My dress zipped up with room to spare, and I had the perfect night in my perfect dress. But it was a hollow victory, coming at a terrible cost. That first experience with crash dieting kicked off a two-decade-long, tangled relationship with my body, self-esteem, and food.

Muscle Power, Mind Power Tip #3:
My Inner Regina George

I was under no illusions. I knew a 90-pound weight loss journey would be hard, especially after spending 20 years failing miserably to lose weight.

My outlook was grim.

I envisioned a future dominated by the word *no*. *No* dessert. *No* drinks out with friends. *No* fun ever again. I imagined choking down gallons of suspicious-looking meal replacement shakes while subjecting myself to endless hours of cardio with Chalene Johnson. Those early 2000s workout DVDs were truly a unique form of self-punishment, weren't they?

My plan felt like a recipe for pure misery, somewhere on par with crossing the Sahara Desert in stilettos. But I was actually wrong about the hard part. It wasn't Chalene or the cheese drawer's siren call that broke me time and time again.

It was the war raging inside my head.

Allow me to formally (re)introduce my inner critic. You remember her, right? She was the charming drill sergeant meticulously calculating my cardio-for-Chardonnay exchange rate a few chapters ago.

We all have a voice inside our heads that loves to analyze (or overanalyze) everything we do. Ideally, our inner critics would be helpful internal guides, like tiny life coaches offering constructive criticism and pointing us toward growth. But give her an unchecked microphone for too long, and your inner critic transforms into a full-blown bully.

Mine was the Regina George of my mind. It felt like the movie *Mean Girls* was playing out in my cranium. Instead of ruling the halls of North Shore High with an arched eyebrow, she was busy terrorizing my thoughts with her perfectly manicured set of claws.

Schoolyard bullies use insults to hurt you, but a rogue inner critic uses flawed patterns of thinking called cognitive distortions. They distort reality by magnifying the negative and minimizing the positive. Think of it like looking at life through a dirty window, with dirt and streaks obscuring the beauty outside. My inner mean girl was a master manipulator and an expert at selective memory. She made sure my failures lingered while my successes vanished into thin air.

When I first started writing this book, I debated whether I wanted to lay this particular piece of my mental chaos bare. For the longest time, I was convinced my inner critic wasn't just your standard-issue negative voice. She was some kind of specially commissioned and uniquely cruel personal tormentor assigned solely to me.

That conviction was incredibly isolating. I rarely tried to explain what I was going through to my support system, because the words would just seize up in my throat. Even surrounded by their love and encouragement, the shame and embarrassment of sounding completely unhinged held me back from sharing the full extent.

Seriously, was anyone else's brain this aggressively mean? Could this level of internal static even be remotely normal?

The answer is the classic (and infuriating), "*Yes... but also no.*"

The "yes" part? Our brains are hardwired with a "negativity bias." Not surprisingly, evolution prioritized survival over self-esteem. So, while our ancestors were busy developing a keen sense of danger, they probably overlooked the small stuff, like successfully foraging for berries, or the incredibly minor advancement of inventing the wheel (which, in their defense, probably didn't seem like a huge deal at the time).

The point is that the brain tends to overanalyze every perceived misstep, while positive experiences slip away like sand through your fingers.

Now for the crucial "no" part. No one deserves to be bullied, not by a "Plastic" in the high school cafeteria plotting your social demise, and certainly not by the resident bully camped out in your own mind. There's no negotiating with bullies, and my inner mean girl was no exception.

I needed to fight back.

But she would prove to be a formidable opponent. If she were a boxer, she'd be the undisputed trash-talking champion, undefeated for over 20 years. Taking her down would mean fighting her punch by punch, even if those punches were aimed squarely at my own insecurities.

This wouldn't be my story if it didn't include the messy, uncomfortable battle with my inner mean girl and her arsenal of cognitive distortions. It raged for years, shaping my beliefs about myself and my ability to succeed. But I also know I'm not alone in this. So many of us wage this silent war against our own minds every single day.

If you're nodding along in solidarity, grateful that it's not just you, or laughing out loud, thinking, "OMG, this girl's a complete nutcase!" I've done my job. A little levity and a sense of shared experience never hurt anyone, right?

Muscle Power, Mind Power Tip #4: The Basics—Sleep, Stress, Hydration, Nutrition, Exercise

When you're trying to figure out how to get healthier or change your body, the health and fitness world throws a lot of flashy promises at you. I've been around the block a few times and seen many trends come and go.

- Fancy supplements? *Check.*
- Over-the-top workout routines? *Check, check.*
- Restrictive diets where you exist on Diet Coke and sadness for weeks on end? *Check, check, check!*

But what made the biggest difference for me and what I truly believe works long-term? The boring but oh-so-important basics. There are five key elements to any successful, sustainable lifestyle change: Sleep, Stress, Hydration, Nutrition, and Exercise.

Are you ready to get practical?

Sleep

When you think about fat loss, sleep probably isn't the first thing that comes to mind. But as it turns out, it plays a much more significant role than I ever imagined.

When you're well-rested, everything feels more manageable. Your mood is brighter, you have more energy, and making healthy choices feels easy. But after I've had even *one* bad night's sleep?

Forget about it. My inner Cookie Monster takes the wheel, and all bets are off. My energy plummets, and the urgent message my body sends me, loud and clear, is: "Give me sleep, or give me *cookies*! Lots and lots of *cookies*!"

Back in the day, I'd drag myself to the gym at the crack of dawn after a few measly hours of sleep, proudly bragging that I traded in a few extra *Zzz*'s for a calorie burn. I learned the hard way that sacrificing sleep for exercise is like trying to fill a leaky bucket. No matter how much effort you pour in, you'll never get the results you want.

The experts say that adults need 7-9 hours of sleep a night. I'm sure you're thinking, like I did, "Tell that to my overflowing inbox and neverending to-do list!" Because I couldn't magically add more hours to my day, I prioritized my sleep hygiene. If I couldn't sleep *more*, I would at least sleep *better*.

Pro Tip #1: I started with the basics, like a consistent bedtime and wake-up time (even on the weekends), a dark and cool room, and a "no screens" policy that comes into effect an hour before bed. These are tiny tweaks, but they can make a measurable difference in your sleep quality.

Stress

Stress isn't always bad. It's a natural part of life, and we need natural stressors like waking up in the morning and exercising to thrive. Short-term (or acute) stress can also be motivating or exhilarating. In my day job, I thrive on the adrenaline rush of an occasional last-minute request or tight deadline.

But stress becomes problematic when those little stressors pile up or when we're hit with a major life event, like a job loss or grief. High levels of chronic stress can throw our bodies out of whack. It can trigger cravings, slow muscle recovery, and increase fat storage, especially around the belly.

As a work-in-progress recovering workaholic (some days more successfully than others), stress is the basic I wrestle with the most. But I've learned a few helpful tricks along the way.

Pro Tip #2: I like to close my eyes and focus on where I'm feeling stress in my body. Most of the time, it's in my neck and shoulders. I take a few deep breaths and imagine the stress melting away as I exhale.

Pro Tip #3: Maintaining a consistent exercise routine helps me manage my stress. The gym is a calming, relaxing place for me, and I always feel more like myself after a workout. Weightlifting, in particular, shifts my focus away from the stressor and toward the present moment. I find it easy to zone out (and stress out) while strolling on the treadmill. But executing a complex lift with perfect form requires all my focus, giving my mind the break it needs.

Pro Tip #4: As much as I love my technology, the endless notifications and "doomscrolling" can feel overwhelming. I like to unplug and do something that makes me feel relaxed and grounded again. I wish I had the time and patience for scented candles, essential oils, and bubble baths, but it's unrealistic for me. A long, hot shower does the trick every time.

Let's face it. Unless you've sworn off all material things and live in a remote mountaintop monastery fully dedicated to quiet contemplation and spiritual practice, feeling Zen 24/7 is an unrealistic expectation. I've found a few tricks to help me manage my stress more effectively, but I'm no guru. Your path to inner peace might look completely different. Explore and experiment so you can discover what brings you back to center.

Hydration

I've always been more of a Diet Coke connoisseur than a water drinker. While there's nothing wrong with consuming artificially sweetened beverages, I wasn't properly hydrated. I was basically a walking raisin. But once I focused on hydration, my workouts improved, my cravings decreased, and even my skin looked better.

It turns out that science agrees with my lived experience. Proper hydration impacts everything from your energy levels and mental clarity to how well your muscles work and even how efficiently you digest that delicious burrito you had for lunch. Conversely, even mild dehydration can reduce energy and slow metabolism, making losing fat harder.

The standard advice is to aim for half your body weight (in pounds) in ounces of water daily. So, if you weigh 150 pounds, your target would be 75 ounces. It might seem like a lot, but your body will thank you. And your skin will probably look fantastic, too!

Pro Tip #5: One of my favorite tricks is to have a glass of water before every meal. This is called habit stacking, where you build a new habit (drinking water) by anchoring it to an existing one (eating). The idea was popularized in the book *Atomic Habits* by James Clear, which you should definitely check out.

Pro Tip #6: Find a water bottle you love and keep it by your side throughout the day. Mine is a cheerful seafoam green mug my brother bought me for Christmas. It makes me smile and reminds me to drink up!

Nutrition

I know firsthand that diving headfirst into restriction mode is tempting when you're fired up to start a health and fitness transformation. You want to cut out sugar, banish bread, and wage war on anything processed, but restriction often backfires in a big way. When I feel deprived, I get the most intense cravings for anything I've deemed "off limits." Before long, I'm elbow-deep in a sleeve of Oreos.

When I shifted my mindset to focus on what I could add to my diet, I found it gentler and more sustainable. The two things I focused on adding were protein and fiber.

Let's start with protein. It's a vital part of many metabolic processes, helping with things like blood sugar regulation, hormone production, and energy expenditure. It also supports a healthy body composition by keeping you full and satisfied. Protein is also the building block of muscle, a metabolically active tissue that burns calories even at rest. Strong muscles improve physical performance and help protect against chronic diseases like Type 2 diabetes and heart disease. Finally, as we age, our ability to synthesize protein declines, making adequate protein intake even more critical for maintaining muscle mass and promoting healthy aging.

Dr. Gabrielle Lyon's book *Forever Strong* cemented in my mind the crucial role of protein in building muscle, and its ripple effects on overall health, metabolic function, and even longevity. She argues that the current protein recommendations are outdated and fall short, advocating for a bare minimum of 30 grams of high-quality protein per meal for optimal health and well-being.

Pro Tip #7: Once I started building my meals around protein, I naturally ate less without the dreaded feeling of deprivation. It was like my body finally felt nourished and chilled out on the cravings. That's also when I started seeing more dramatic changes in my physique, because I was building more muscle, which made me look less squishy and more defined.

The second thing I'd do is prioritize fiber.

I used to think of fruits and vegetables as optional side dishes, afterthoughts on my plate. But I've learned that they're crucial for a healthy diet. They provide essential vitamins, minerals, and antioxidants, and the added bulk keeps me fuller for longer. Fiber helps slow digestion and keeps things moving smoothly through your system. It also helps regulate blood sugar levels, which can help curb cravings and prevent overeating. Plus, a high-fiber diet is excellent for gut health, which is linked to all sorts of benefits, like improved mood and a stronger immune system.

The standard advice is to eat 14 grams of fiber per 1,000 calories consumed. So, for a 150-pound woman, a good place to start is

25-30 grams per day. But there isn't really a downside to aiming higher!

Pro Tip #8: I treat myself like a toddler and hide my vegetables. I add spinach to my scrambled eggs or make my mac and cheese a little heartier with pureed cauliflower or butternut squash. You can barely even taste it, and you get the benefit of an added nutritional boost.

Exercise

When people hear I've lost a significant amount of weight through lifestyle change, the questions they ask me rarely have anything to do with how often I work out or what I eat for breakfast. Instead, it's almost always: "Lisa, how did you stay so *motivated* to lose 90 pounds?" or "Seriously, where do you find the *willpower* to drag yourself to the gym so regularly?"

I understand why. We all know exercise is good for us. It has a permanent place on our list of "should dos," right alongside "eat more vegetables" and "call your mom more often." But the real conversation, the one that comes up time and again in my story, is about the gap between knowing something is good for you and consistently doing it. The negotiation between our best intentions and our actions is a struggle most of us know intimately.

This battle is so universal because our brains run on ancient software, essentially "Survival 1.0." We're meant to prioritize immediate comfort, seek out easy energy, and conserve precious resources, not enthusiastically sign up for an hour of lunges and push-ups that promise vague, intangible benefits somewhere down the road. Exercise means upfront effort for delayed gratification, which reliably (and justifiably) prompts a "Hard pass!" from our primal brains.

I'm sure that on some level, the people asking me those questions about my motivation and willpower knew I wasn't about to reveal a secret strategy or life-altering hack that I was gatekeeping. But my answer still threw them for a loop.

I don't rely on either one.

Relying on motivation and willpower is why so many New Year's resolutions are abandoned come the beginning of February. Constantly trying to strong-arm yourself into exercising using sheer willpower is exhausting, and chasing motivation leaves you with nothing more than your good intentions and probably a new pair of unused gym sneakers. There are ways to temporarily boost motivation and willpower (and we could absolutely dedicate a chapter or two to these tactics), but I'd rather talk about something far more reliable that gives a significant and enduring return on your effort.

Consistent action.

That's the unglamorous, often uncelebrated, but unbelievably effective truth.

BJ Fogg, author of the book *Tiny Habits*, has this brilliant way of explaining how to use consistent action to build lasting habits. His advice is to start so ridiculously small it feels almost silly, like doing a single push-up a day while your coffee brews. Now, obviously, that one push-up won't grant you Michelle Obama arms overnight. Its genius is in making the act of starting so unbelievably easy and non-threatening that it outsmarts your brain's "Survival 1.0" software, and you end up building a new habit without the fight.

This is where it really gets good.

Once you've started something (because your brain barely notices you tricking it into action), you're much more likely to keep going. If you're already on the floor for your token push-up, what's one more? Or two? If you've already laced up your sneakers and walked for 5 minutes, suddenly another 5 doesn't seem as daunting. Every small "yes" makes the next "yes" easier and quiets that urge to quit. This is how consistency (not some burst of here-today-gone-tomorrow motivation or a short-lived bout of white-knuckled willpower) will reliably get you moving, build your strength, increase your energy, and deliver all those incredible benefits exercise promises.

Pro Tip #9: Start by finding some form of movement you enjoy (or, at the absolute minimum, tolerate). Commit to small, consistent actions until you've built momentum, and keep going until the momentum translates that new behavior into an ingrained, almost effortless, habit.

As we dig deeper into my story, I'll share exactly how I unknowingly put this whole "start tiny, build momentum, and stay consistent" strategy to work, transforming myself from an on-again-off-again (honestly, mostly off-again) elliptical devotee into someone who actually uses the squat rack.

The Power of the (Actually Doable) Basics

My legs are my biggest insecurity. That's where I carried most of my weight, and despite years of training and significant fat loss, they still don't look the way I hoped they would. If I could buy a magic pill and instantly rock Tina Turner's iconic legs (at any age!), I'd be the first in line, yelling, "Take my money!"

But that level of celebrity fabulousness is often the result of a combination of superior genetics, focused dedication, ultra-specific training, meticulously controlled nutrition, an entourage team of stylists, and perfect lighting.

For most of us, that's an unrealistic, unattainable ideal.

In chasing those out-of-reach "ideal" results, many of us get suckered into what we believe are "optimal" plans. These plans promise the quickest, most dramatic transformations, usually involving super-detailed, cutting-edge, ridiculously complicated strategies. Flashy "optimal" approaches aren't just unsustainable, they encourage us to overlook the quiet power of the basics. If I'd only understood that the basics would effectively get me 80% of the way to my goals, I would have started there much sooner.

The path to feeling strong, capable, and genuinely good in your own skin is rarely paved with "optimal" intentions. It's almost always built on a foundational approach, constructed brick by brick through the consistent mastery of the unsexy but essential basics, the habits you can actually live with, day in and day out.

CHAPTER 2

My Battle with Binge Eating Disorder

I remember my high school graduation like it was yesterday.

There I was in my shimmering crimson satin gown, feeling like the main character in my very own coming-of-age movie. Confidence radiated from me as I danced the night away, surrounded by friends who felt like family. We were invincible, ready to take on the world. With my diploma in hand and a bright smile on my face, I was brimming with optimism about the future. It was a night of endless possibilities, friendships that felt like they'd last a lifetime, and the exhilarating feeling that I could achieve anything I set my mind to.

But life after graduation didn't go as planned. Those fragile early adult years were some of the hardest I've ever faced. There were moments when I felt lost, overwhelmed, and alone, desperately seeking comfort and connection in a world that felt increasingly hostile and indifferent.

While I wouldn't wish those experiences on anyone, they taught me valuable lessons about strength and vulnerability. They shaped me into the person I am today. But at the time, it was impossible for me to appreciate the hardships I was facing for the wisdom they were imparting.

Struggle shapes us in many different ways. While some people face challenges by seeking support, tackling problems head-on, or breaking down big issues into manageable chunks, others turn to unhelpful or even harmful coping mechanisms.

My harmful coping mechanism was food.

I've often asked myself *why*. *Why* did I respond the way I did in the face of adversity? *Why* did food become my comfort, my escape from stress? *Why* was it my go-to strategy for dealing with uncomfortable feelings instead of literally anything else?

With the clarity of hindsight, I can see how my life experiences subtly nudged me in that direction. I have so many happy memories tied to food, like cozy family dinners, the thrill of picking out my favorite snacks for movie night, or the epic ice cream sundae feasts my mom would lovingly plan for my brother and me, complete with every topping imaginable. Food meant happy times, connection, and love. It felt like being wrapped in a big, warm hug.

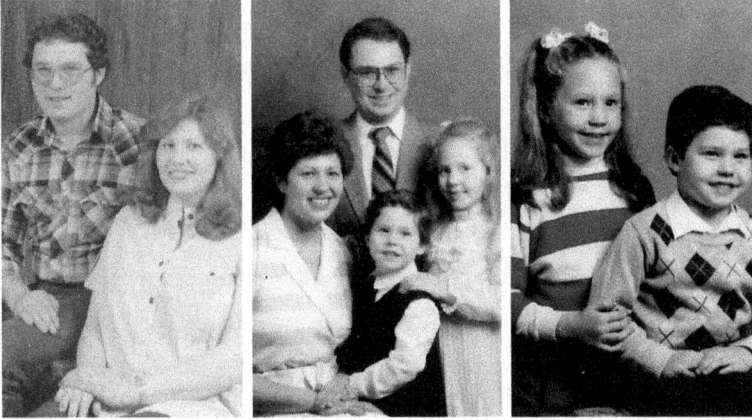

The Labre Family—Gerry, Donna, Lisa, and Brent.

When my life felt out of control, food was a comfort that made sense, because it brought me back to a time when I felt safe. As I increasingly relied on food to regulate my emotions and deal with my problems, I lost sight of healthier coping mechanisms, like journaling, talking to a friend, or taking a walk. While eating had once been about nourishment, joy, and connection with my loved ones, without my awareness, it had subtly shifted into an escape. Every bite was a mini-vacation from the problems I wasn't ready to face.

I can still remember every detail of my first binge-eating episode. This was the moment I crossed the line into a full-blown eating disorder.

In the summer of 2004, I took a leap of faith. I moved to a bigger city, chasing a new job opportunity and hoping to turn my long-distance relationship into something real. He was a great guy, but he was wrestling with his own demons and emotionally unavailable. Living together only highlighted the vast emotional distance between us, and my loneliness was amplified by being so far from my family.

To top it all off, I absolutely despised my job. The call center I worked in was an introvert's worst nightmare, with its constant pressure to hit sales targets and the endless stream of superficial client interactions. I was always talking but never connecting with anyone. I left work every day feeling mentally and physically drained.

One year later, in the summer of 2005, the relationship predictably came to an end. With a heavy heart, I found a tiny studio apartment and faced the reality of living alone for the first time. My ever-supportive parents drove six hours from my hometown to spend the weekend celebrating my twenty-fifth birthday while helping me find furniture and settle in. I was grateful to have the comfort of family as I tried to piece my broken heart back together and adjust to yet another new chapter in my life.

But the weekend ended, and my folks had to go home and get back to their lives. After they left, the silence in my apartment was more than I could handle. I should have been out with friends, laughing and celebrating. Instead, loneliness hit hard. Desperate for a distraction, I decided to treat myself to a massive feast.

Like the thousands of binges that would follow, this one was meticulously planned and involved different foods. I wanted some form of pure sugar (candies), some combination of sugar and fat (ice cream), a pastry (cookies, donuts, or snack cakes), something crunchy (chips), and something with both fat and salt (burgers and fries, or pizza). That day, I picked up six donuts, a pint of ice cream, a family-sized bag of chips, and some gummy bears. Then, I added a double cheeseburger, fries, and a Diet Coke. It made no logical sense, of course, but the diet soda somehow took the edge off the guilt I was feeling for the calorie-dense meal I was about to consume.

The donuts were melt-in-your-mouth soft and sweet. The chips crunched loudly as I stuffed them into my mouth, one handful after another. The fries burned the back of my throat with their salty, vinegary goodness. The cheeseburger was greasy, leaving a satisfyingly cheesy film in my mouth. The ice cream was cold and creamy, numbing my senses as I ate spoonful after spoonful.

Eating different flavors and textures overrides the body's natural fullness cues, which are elegantly designed to gently make us aware of when we've had enough to eat. It makes perfect sense. Think about what happens when you go to a restaurant for dinner. You polish off your main course, feeling full as you push your plate away, confident you can't eat another bite. But then, the dessert menu arrives. Suddenly, you're thinking, "I could definitely go for something sweet!" It's the "dessert stomach" or "hollow leg" paradox in action.

With the TV blaring in the background in an attempt to drown out the silence, I lost myself in eating. I consumed every last crumb of that junk food feast, devouring thousands of calories in a daze as I tried to use food to fill an emotional void, something it was never meant to do.

There was no joy in that first binge or any of the others that would follow. There was only desperation as I used food to build a wall between myself and the world.

Sometimes, logic would peek through in the middle of a binge, and I'd try to stop myself by throwing away whatever food was left. I'd feel a little better, like I'd momentarily regained control. But it never lasted. Before I knew it, I was digging through the trash to rescue the food I'd just thrown away. I felt disgusted with myself and understood this wasn't normal behavior around food.

The drive to binge was overwhelmingly powerful, a desperate need to numb myself. This need quickly turned eating from a coping mechanism into a full-blown emotional anesthetic. I wanted that temporary peace so badly that it felt like the only thing that mattered. Inevitably, the effects of the anesthetic would wear off moments after the last bite was swallowed, and I was left to face the tangled mess of my feelings, now exacerbated by the physical discomfort and the shame of overeating.

The next few years were a blur of heartache and turmoil. Throughout all of this, my binge eating was simultaneously my only coping mechanism and a personal failure that chipped away at my self-esteem. The number on the scale climbed relentlessly, trapping me in a dangerous cycle of binging and extreme dieting. In quiet moments of desperate honesty, I would consider reaching out to someone for help. Deep down, I knew this was a cycle I couldn't break alone. Finally, after two years of secretly battling an eating disorder, I reached out to my family doctor as the first tentative step on a long and difficult journey toward recovery.

In 2007, I was formally diagnosed with Binge Eating Disorder (BED). I felt relieved when the struggle I'd been wrestling with for so long was finally given a name. BED is a serious condition characterized by episodes of eating large amounts of food very quickly, to the point of discomfort, followed by feelings of loss of control, shame, distress, and guilt. It's more common than you might think and can have a devastating impact on your physical and mental health.

I thought receiving that diagnosis would flip a switch in my mind and change everything, but it didn't. I was still stuck, a frustrating reminder that knowing better rarely translates to doing better automatically. We all know someone who, despite a life-altering diagnosis like heart disease or diabetes, can't seem to make the lifestyle changes that would improve their health. I knew I was hurting myself, but that wasn't enough to make a change. Even with a dangerous and highly self-destructive condition, I returned to the only source of comfort I knew when difficult emotions hit.

By my early thirties, binge eating had become my default response to any negative emotion. Fear, anxiety, anger, stress, boredom, or even just feeling tired, it all felt like a bottomless pit of hunger to me. But this wasn't the kind of hunger you could satisfy with a sandwich. It would build from a low hum of anxiety into an agitated emptiness, an urgent, almost frantic need for anything to make the discomfort stop. It was relentless and visceral, like my heart was silently screaming, pleading for relief. Instead of self-soothing and giving my heart the comfort or escape from the loneliness it was begging for, I muffled its screams with empty calories. I ate chocolate bars, chips, or candy, anything to numb the pain.

As the years went on, I battled depression, navigated family and financial struggles, and endured the pain of a failed marriage. Then, I lost my dad. Like any father-daughter relationship, it was sometimes complicated but always filled with a fierce, unmistakable love that was uniquely ours. His sudden death left a gaping hole in my life. There were so many things left unsaid and so many questions left unanswered. I'm grateful he made his exit from this world quickly and without pain, but that knowledge did little to ease the overwhelming grief I felt.

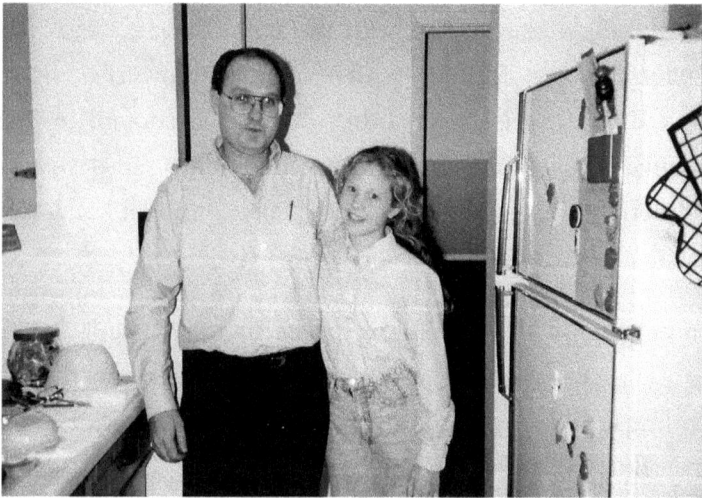

Gerry "Ger-Ber" Labre, 1954-2015.
I love you and miss you every day, Dad.

By that point, my binging was so ingrained in my life that I started binging when I felt anything at all, even positive emotions. My brain felt broken, like I couldn't tell the difference between my feelings any longer. Was I upset? Irritated? Frustrated? Happy? Anxious? Lonely? Joyful? Overwhelmed? Who knows! I certainly didn't.

The only circuit remaining was horrifyingly simple: Feelings = hamburger.

The ritual of grabbing my "go-to" binge foods had become almost automatic, a well-worn path I could navigate on autopilot. One minute, I was driving home from work on a Tuesday night and the next, I was in my living room with a cheeseburger in my lap, chocolate on my fingers, and Cheeto dust in my hair, with no memory of how I got there. The whole thing was objectively absurd, but there's nothing objective about binge eating. It was just my reality.

I remember one particularly mortifying incident. I'd stopped at the pharmacy to pick up a prescription. While I waited, I mindlessly wandered into the snack food section. It was like muscle memory kicked in as my hands frantically reached for chips, candy, and chocolate in a trance-like state. With my arms piled high with my haul, I rounded the corner and nearly collided with a former colleague who hadn't seen me since my eating had spiraled out of control. Reality knocked me out of my trance, and embarrassment quickly kicked in. I frantically dumped everything into a nearby bin and bolted out of the store, leaving my prescription behind. To this day, I don't know if she even recognized me, but the humiliation I felt in that moment is something I won't forget.

The toll binge eating had on my physical health was undeniable. Years of disordered eating led to a weight gain of over 100 pounds and a cascade of health issues. The emotional toll was equally devastating. I had no faith that change was possible, and I was convinced I was destined to live a life defined by my struggle with food. Every attempt at change felt futile, like fighting an invisible enemy that was always one step ahead.

Today, I see my struggles and setbacks as necessary parts of the learning process. Even the most successful people will tell you they have a graveyard full of "almosts" and "not quites" in their past. I tried different approaches, but my instincts, wired for the familiar, fought back fiercely. Slipping back into old patterns was depressingly easy. But actually breaking those cycles? That felt impossible.

For twelve long years after my diagnosis, I felt trapped, powerless to create any real change.

Muscle Power, Mind Power Tip #5:
Beyond Binge Eating

While I'm sharing my experience and the strategies that helped me, they should not replace professional medical advice and support. Seeking guidance from qualified specialists is essential for addressing any eating disorder. Think of this as a resource guide to accompany you on your journey, not a substitute for expert care.

At first, I thought that understanding my diagnosis would cure my binge eating. But that was just the tip of the iceberg. As I explored the psychology behind my diagnosis, I gradually discovered ideas and tools that shed light on my struggle. I incorporated them with patience and persistence into my life, making subtle yet significant changes to my habits and patterns. Eventually, these incremental shifts accumulated, weakening the grip of the binge eating cycle and allowing me to take my first tentative steps toward recovery.

The first thing that clicked for me was that binge eating, like any habit, follows a predictable pattern. In the book *The Power of Habit*, author Charles Duhigg breaks this down into a three-part loop:

- *Trigger*: The cue that initiates the habit. My triggers were feelings like stress, anxiety, boredom, or loneliness.
- *Action*: The behavior itself. For me, that was binge eating.

- *Reward*: The payoff that tells your brain to do it again. My reward was a temporary feeling of relief from discomfort.

Understanding the habit loop was a step in the right direction, but it didn't completely solve the problem. I still had to figure out how to break the loop, a battle that put my impulsive and rational selves at odds with one another.

I love the way Jonathan Haidt's book, *The Happiness Hypothesis*, explains the struggle between our impulsive and rational selves with a metaphor of an elephant and its rider. The elephant represents the older, more instinctive part of our brain, driven by emotions and seeking instant gratification. It's the part of us that craves that sugary treat or wants to hit the snooze button. The rider is our rational brain. This part understands long-term consequences and tries to steer us toward actions that align with our goals.

As Haidt explains, when triggered with a familiar cue, the elephant will take off, charging down its well-worn path. The rider can have all the good intentions in the world, but there isn't much she can do to control the powerful, emotional elephant.

With this information, I thought I had it all figured out. My plan was to avoid or eliminate my triggers to prevent binges before they even started. It didn't take long for that simple plan to fall apart. Some triggers were relatively easy to avoid. For example, if I didn't buy the Oreos in the first place, they weren't in my house to eat. But how was I supposed to avoid the triggers that came with being a human, like work stress, family drama, or a lack of sleep?

Thanks to another resource, I shifted my focus from managing my triggers to managing how I reacted to them. Josh Hillis' book, *Lean and Strong: Eating Skills, Psychology, and Workouts*, gave me new tools to help me manage my urges to binge.

The first is a simple pause. When a craving hits, I set a ten-minute timer instead of immediately giving in. During that time, I use body-focused techniques to ground myself, like breathwork and paying close attention to the physical sensations related to the craving. Or, I distract myself with work, an errand, or something fun like a hobby. After the timer runs out, I check in with myself. True hunger? I eat. Still feeling the urge to binge? I binge, free of guilt and shame. More often than not, the pause calms my inner elephant, allowing my rational brain to catch up and bring my goals back into focus.

The second tool, closely linked to the first, is an idea called "urge surfing." Hillis accurately describes the experience of a craving like a wave that builds until it peaks and eventually subsides. "Urge surfing" is the skill of riding out the wave. Reminding myself that cravings don't last can sometimes be enough to keep me from acting on them. Awareness makes me feel like the ultimate surfer girl, riding the wave without wiping out.

My favorite concept from Hillis' book is the idea of aligning food choices with values, which means learning to say "yes" to food when it aligns with your values and "no" when it doesn't. For example, there's a big difference between sharing a slice of cheesecake with your partner on date night because it nourishes your connection (and your soul!) and demolishing an entire cheesecake solo on a Friday night because you're bored and lonely.

My understanding of binge eating shifted yet again when I encountered Glenn Livingston's unconventional and controversial book, initially titled *Never Binge Again* (now updated to *Defeat Your Cravings*). He suggests treating the craving brain as a separate entity, as something that isn't even a part of you. He refers to the craving brain as a "pig" that is undeserving of empathy and incapable of negotiation. He also suggests de-romanticizing binge foods by calling them "slop," a term he uses to strip them of their power and allure.

Initially, I found his approach obnoxious and it didn't resonate with me at all. But there was one thing that *did* make sense. Livingston's method involves creating strict rules about what you "always" or "never" do. In general, I don't believe that this type of "all-or-nothing" thinking is helpful. But there is a specific instance where it worked for me.

I occasionally enjoy processed foods like peanut butter cups and movie popcorn, and cutting them out of my life is unrealistic. But these foods also trigger binges. Recognizing that my binge eating only happened when I was alone, I made one rule: "I *never* eat ultra-processed, highly palatable food *alone*."

I maintain this rule to this day.

Obviously, I'm just scratching the surface of what these folks have taught me, so if my brief summary has sparked your interest, I would encourage you to seek out these resources to get the full picture.

I know I sound like a broken record. Still, I can't emphasize this enough. These strategies have been transformative for me, and I genuinely hope they will be for you, too. But please, don't go through this by yourself. I remember the countless hours poring over books and scouring the internet, feeling isolated and desperate for answers.

It breaks my heart to think of you doing the same.

There are caring, compassionate people out there who understand what you're going through and are ready to support you on your journey to recovery.

Reach out. You're not alone.

Muscle Power, Mind Power Tip #6: Emotional Eating

Naively, I assumed that as I progressed in my recovery from BED, my emotional connection to food would simply vanish. I learned, however, that an emotional eater isn't necessarily a binge eater, and the distinction between the two is far more nuanced than I thought. Even as my actions no longer met the clinical definition of BED, I was still stuck because my emotions were still a powerful trigger, and food was still the best coping strategy I had.

Let me explain my relationship with food and emotional eating with a funny story from my childhood.

I inherited a major fear of bees from my dad. When he was young, he had a nasty run-in with a swarm, and even in adulthood, the sight of a single bee would send him into a full-blown panic.

My mom loves to tell the story of one beautiful summer afternoon when she sent my dad and me outside to play while she cooked dinner. The sun was shining, birds were chirping, and my dad and I should have been frolicking gleefully in the backyard. But when my mom opened the back door to call us in for dinner, she couldn't believe what she saw.

The two of us were huddled under my overturned bright green, frog-shaped, child-sized swimming pool.

Why, you ask? Good question!

We'd spotted a lone bee buzzing around the yard.

I'm sure the bee was just peacefully going about its honey-making business. But to us, it was on a hostile attack mission, dive-bombing us at every chance. Until she did a full-on bee sweep to confirm that the coast was clear, we wouldn't consider emerging from our plastic amphibian sanctuary.

I used to treat my emotions like my dad and I treated bees. They were something to be avoided at all costs. Uncomfortable feelings? Nope, I'm not dealing with those! Instead, I'd do anything to numb them out, often turning to food for comfort.

Rationally, I understood that a pint of Ben & Jerry's wouldn't solve my problems or that a bag of chips wouldn't mend my broken heart. But in the moment when those emotions came buzzing around, logic would take a backseat. Avoiding my feelings strengthened them instead of making them disappear. Each unprocessed emotion was like another bee in an ever-growing hive, buzzing louder and louder until I was overwhelmed by the swarm.

Unless you're allergic, or you've been stung by some deadly creature from the depths of the Australian Outback, the anticipation of a sting is usually worse than the sting itself.

Feelings work the same way. Unless you're dealing with the kind of mental or emotional distress that demands professional intervention, the fear of a feeling is often more painful than the feeling itself. Allowing yourself to feel those uncomfortable emotions can be scary, but it's often not as bad as you imagine.

Eventually, it fades as you process and move through the experience, just like an itchy sting heals over time.

There's no denying the powerful connection between food and our emotions, and it's not always a bad thing. It's woven into so many parts of our lives, from our happiest memories and the ways we celebrate to the comfort we seek in heartache. Whenever I eat my mom's cooking, it tastes like love, nostalgia, and happy childhood memories.

But there's a fine line between enjoying an occasional indulgence and using food as a crutch. When I notice myself consistently reaching for ice cream instead of dealing with difficult emotions, I recognize that it's time to reassess my relationship with Ben & Jerry and consider that it might be keeping me stuck instead of helping me heal.

Approaching unpleasant feelings with curiosity and kindness and observing my emotions as they buzz around me still feels uncomfortable. Sometimes they sting a little, sometimes a lot. Most of the time, they eventually just buzz away. No matter how it plays out, I always feel stronger for facing them head-on instead of hiding under a frog-shaped pool.

CHAPTER 3

The Last False Start

It was early August 2019, a few weeks before my thirty-ninth birthday. A friend and I were catching up over dinner at a cute, cozy restaurant. Surrounded by lively chatter, clinking glasses, and delicious food, we were having a great time.

As the evening progressed and the wine flowed, nature called. The tables were placed a little too close, and the patrons were packed in like sardines. Sitting with my back to the wall and fellow diners to my left and right, I faced the dilemma of extracting myself from my cramped surroundings. How do I get out? Do I turn my front or my back to the neighboring table?

My situation was giving *Fight Club* vibes, like that scene on the airplane where Tyler Durden poses the same question. I swear I heard someone say, "You are not your skinny jeans," as I contemplated the social implications of my exit strategy.

It's always a gamble, but as Durden did, I opted for the rear, hoping to minimize accidental contact with strangers. As I wiggled and shimmied my way out, disaster struck. My butt bumped a glass, sending a cascade of red wine across the table and onto the woman sitting next to me. Mortified, I apologized profusely, offering to pay for her dry cleaning as I frantically dabbed at the mess with my napkin. She was so much more gracious than I would have been in her situation, assuring me it was an accident.

Sure, a simple accident in a crowded restaurant could have happened to anyone. But it happened to *me*, and my inner mean girl wouldn't let me off the hook. "Maybe if you hadn't raided the bread basket," she cackled, "your *giant ass* wouldn't have knocked over that wine!"

Try as I might, I couldn't shake it off, and the embarrassment lingered. The scene replayed in my mind, every detail exaggerated by my insecurities. Lost in thought as I wandered home, I caught a glimpse of my reflection in a brightly lit shop window, and it stopped me dead in my tracks. I didn't recognize the woman staring back at me.

"When did I get so... *round*?" I thought to myself.

The shop window reflection of my too-tight jeans, straining against my waistline, confirmed a truth I had been desperately avoiding. I had gained weight. *Again.*

The following day, I walked into the bathroom, and there it was. The scale gleamed menacingly at me from the corner of the room. I swear it was mocking me. I gingerly placed a toe on the corner, then quickly yanked it back. "*Why me?*" I wailed to the uncaring bathroom tiles with a dramatic sigh. "Haven't I suffered enough? Is there no escape from your tyranny?" But the scale remained silent, its digital display blinking innocently. With a frustrated groan, I grabbed the nearest towel and flung it over the scale.

Out of sight, out of mind, right?

Then, I plunged headfirst into another punishing "restrict and sacrifice" diet, coupled with a shiny new gym membership. Surely, *this time*, sheer willpower and self-flagellation would work.

After two weeks of a calorie-sparse diet and the kind of cardio-intense sessions that would make even the meanest, toughest drill sergeant weep for mercy, I was a hangry, exhausted, caffeine-fueled mess. But the *discipline* I had shown gave me just enough courage to face the enemy.

I hesitantly approached the mound of towels steadily accumulating in the corner of my bathroom. With a trembling hand, I pulled them away, and uncovered the scale. It was a simple household object, oblivious to the dread it inspired and its power over my emotions. Reluctantly, I stripped down and muttered a prayer to the weight loss gods.

"Please, *please* let it be lower. I really need a win here. *Just…this… once.*"

I closed my eyes, braced myself, and stepped on. Holding my breath, I slowly opened one eye, peeking through a sliver of lashes. The numbers glared back at me with cold indifference.

Weight: *273 lbs*
Body Fat: 56%

"What the *actual fuck*?!" I shrieked, recoiling from the scale like it had burned me. "How can someone be *more than half fat*? This can't be happening."

The room started to spin, and my stomach was in knots. Even after two weeks of "restrict and sacrifice," that was the highest number I had ever seen on the scale.

Two hundred and seventy-three.

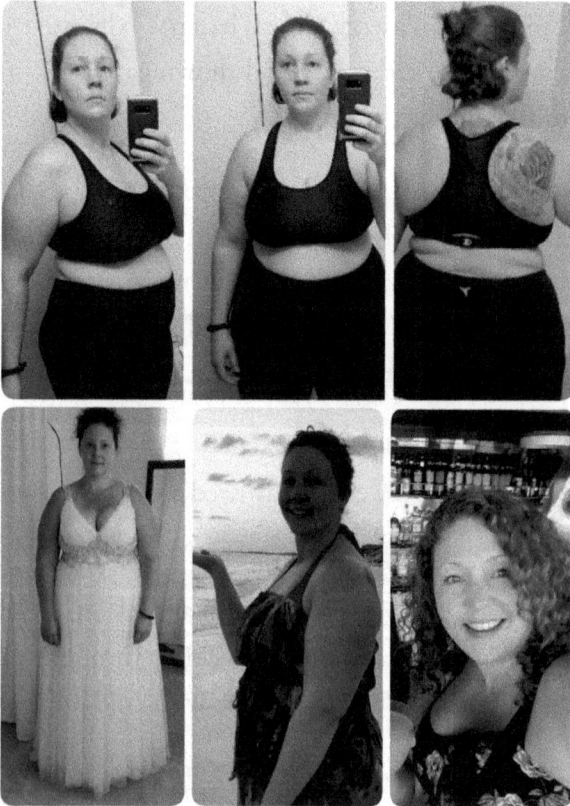

My "before" pictures.

The sickness and disgust I felt took me back to a devastating morning years prior when the scale had flashed 200 pounds for the first time. Back then, I had sobbed, raged, and vowed to never, *ever*, see that number again. Now, here I was, surpassing that long-forgotten promise and hurtling toward 300 pounds.

My inner mean girl was never one to miss a chance to kick me while I was down. She chimed in with a venomous, "See? I told you so. You're a massive, disgusting failure. Just give up already because you'll *never* change."

Years of binging, emotional eating, yo-yo dieting, and general body neglect had culminated in this soul-crushing moment. The number on the scale that day measured so much more than the weight of my body. It measured the weight of a lifetime of broken promises, missed opportunities, and dreams deferred. It was the weight of fun social events skipped, connections with friends lost, and personal and professional growth sacrificed at the altar of insecurity. My life, my dreams, and my social circle had all shrunk as my body expanded.

This was my life, suffocating under the oppressive weight of obesity.

My "restrict and sacrifice" mentality once again disintegrated. The couch called my name, pizza promised instant gratification, and Ben & Jerry offered comfort and solace. I couldn't resist. I retreated back into my familiar old habits as binge eating and Netflix replaced my salads and gym visits.

I thought seeing my highest weight ever and the ensuing downward spiral were my biggest problems. It felt like rock bottom, but as it turns out, I still had a long way to fall. While I was busy fixating on the numbers on the scale, a Category 5 crisis was brewing in my personal life. I couldn't see that within months, my entire world would fall apart.

Let's start with my career. It had become a soul-sucking purgatory, a mind-numbing daily routine that drained every ounce of energy, enthusiasm, and joy from my existence. I woke up feeling like I was wading through quicksand, trudging through the motions, disconnected and numb. When I finally dragged myself home after work, I had nothing left to give. Each day melted into the next in a monotonous blur of exhaustion and disillusionment.

Then there was my strained marriage. My husband and I started our relationship as two souls seeking refuge in each other during particularly tough times. We lovingly supported each other through some of our worst moments. But as the years passed and the dust finally settled in our lives, the cracks in our foundation started to show. We couldn't communicate or see eye-to-eye on even the simplest things, and the word "compromise" was conspicuously absent from our vocabularies. Staring blankly at one another from opposite sides of the couch only five years after the day we started dating and one year after we said "I do," it had become painfully clear that we had different values. Despite our best intentions and deep affection for one another, we were fundamentally incompatible and hopelessly mismatched.

On top of everything, I hadn't processed my grief over the loss of my dad a few years earlier. I wasn't a stranger to loss, but the death of my father hit on an entirely different level. My dad was a firm believer in the value of education, so rather than dealing with my pain in a healthy way, I channeled it into post-graduate studies. I thought if I made him proud, I'd somehow honor his memory. But all I had done was delay the inevitable by shoving my feelings down.

That's the strange thing about being human. We can carry so much for so long, right up until the moment we can't. And it's never the biggest burdens that finally break us. Seeing 273 pounds on the scale was a blow, but it barely registered against the crushing, invisible weight of everything I carried. It was from that place, feeling like I couldn't fall any lower and I had nothing left to lose, that I somehow managed to make four decisions that would, against all odds, lay the foundation for lasting change.

Decision #1: The Pickup Truck Getaway

I asked my husband for a divorce.

In a misguided attempt to save money, we tried the whole "live together while selling our condo" thing. It was a disaster of epic proportions, a masterclass in how *not* to handle a separation. The tension between us escalated quickly, and I had to get out for the sake of my sanity (not to mention *any* chance of an amicable split). Like *yesterday*.

But picking up the pieces of your life and walking away isn't as easy as they make it sound in a country song. I needed backup. So I called my brother, the one person I knew would have my back, no questions asked, no judgment passed.

Under the cover of darkness, he pulled up to my building in his white pickup truck like a modern-day hero coming to the rescue.

Strategically parked at the curb under my second-floor condo, he barely had time to kill the engine before I was heaving bags filled with my life—clothes, shoes, that random shampoo bottle—out the patio door and into the back of his truck. Anything that didn't make the airborne journey that night was left behind.

Sadly, that included my dignity.

In less than five minutes, the truck was loaded, and we were peeling away, leaving behind a trail of emotional wreckage.

Even if the relationship had run its course, I regret how it all went down. My ex-husband is a good man who deserved better than that brutal ending, swift and unceremonious. It must have looked like a scene ripped straight from a reality TV show to my unsuspecting neighbors. But more than that, I can only imagine how it must have felt to him, watching what he thought would be his future peeling away in the cover of night in a white pickup truck.

I'm self-aware enough to see the wreckage I left behind and the pain I inflicted. I have to laugh at the sheer absurdity of it all, but that moment was one of pure desperation. I knew I wasn't in the right place in my life, and I had to do something. It was a harsh lesson learned with profound regret about the lengths we'll go to when we feel we have no other choice, even when it means hurting others.

Decision #2: When Life Gives You Roaches...

In an unexpected twist of fate (and a desperate attempt to avoid financial ruin), my brother and I decided to become roommates.

We were two siblings in our late thirties, each with their own emotional baggage and quirks, crammed into a shoebox of a two-bedroom apartment. It could have been the script for a sitcom, and some days, it honestly felt like it was.

Our budget-friendly apartment wasn't the pinnacle of luxury living. It was "cozy" in the most generous sense, where the occasional six-legged visitor was considered part of the rent. I could write another book with stories about our shady landlord, the comically intrusive upstairs neighbors, and the persistent cockroach problem that even our most valiant Raid campaigns couldn't defeat.

But none of that mattered.

Even though I was broke, unemployed and navigating a mental health crisis while living in a roach motel run by a slumlord with nosy neighbors, it was a vast improvement over the emotional turmoil I left behind. It was the clean slate I needed and a chance to rebuild my life on my terms.

Decision #3: The Mid-Life Crisis

Next, I did the unthinkable. I confidently handed in my resignation letter and walked out the door. It was a confidence I hadn't earned though, because I had no backup plan.

My loved ones were understandably concerned. From the outside, it looked like a textbook midlife crisis, complete with impulsive decision-making and a reckless disregard for financial security. To be fair, they weren't entirely off base. I was ditching a stable career with benefits and a pension, the holy grail of middle-class security. But from my perspective, I was escaping a black hole of misery cleverly disguised as a respectable career.

I joined the public service with the hope of making a difference. Instead, I was trapped in a bureaucratic nightmare of endless paperwork, mind-numbing meetings, and a soul-crushing lack of purpose. My doctor diagnosed me with burnout, a truth that felt like it barely scratched the surface of the full-blown existential crisis I was living through. I was questioning everything I thought I knew about myself, my career, and my place in the world.

Walking away from that job must have looked like an act of sheer lunacy. But for me, it was the only sane choice left. It was a defiant middle finger to the soul-sucking grind, a desperate grasp for a life that felt authentically mine. It marked the beginning of a journey toward reclaiming my life and my identity.

This brings me to the last of my four life-changing decisions. The first three set the stage, but it was this choice that led to the most meaningful action I had ever taken toward improving my physical and mental health.

This is where my story begins.

Muscle Power, Mind Power Tip #7: The Art of Not Freaking Out

Remember that fateful morning when I hesitantly stepped onto the scale, eyes squeezed shut, praying for a miracle? Instead of the heavens parting to reveal a number I could live with, what glared back at me was 273 pounds, 56 percent body fat. So, less divine gift, more statistical slap in the face. That wasn't my finest moment. In fact, it triggered a full-blown meltdown of near-epic proportions.

It didn't take long for my inner mean girl, with her tiny, blackened heart, to set up camp at the bottom of my shame spiral with a director's chair and a megaphone.

"Well, well, well… Look what we have here!" she drawled. "273 pounds!" Pausing for dramatic effect, she adjusted her tiara. "You're clearly not cut out for this whole *healthy lifestyle* thing. Just accept your fate as a professional couch potato and order a pizza. Extra large, extra cheese. You can't button up your jeans anyway, so what's the point?"

She had a point about the jeans, but it still felt a little harsh.

Because my self-worth was so tied up in my weight, the scale dealt a devastating blow that day. But did it warrant the tsunami of self-loathing that followed?

Absolutely not.

We're all guilty of turning tiny setbacks into near-apocalyptic events. This particular brand of cognitive distortion is called catastrophizing. It's the art of transforming a molehill into a mountain of misery. One missed workout becomes a permanent hiatus from the gym, and one dietary misstep becomes a junk food marathon. When you think about it, this behavior is like noticing your bathroom faucet is leaking, and instead of replacing the gasket, you decide to burn the whole house down. You see one minor issue, and your mind convinces you it's beyond repair, so you give up on fixing it altogether.

The inherent irrationality of catastrophizing is why it's such a progress killer. Why bother trying if you're already convinced you're doomed to fail? It's a self-fulfilling prophecy, a cycle in which negativity fuels inaction, and inaction reinforces negativity.

Being your own worst enemy is exhausting. The constant mental battle left me feeling defeated before I even started. I craved ease and grace, and a desire to treat myself with the same kindness I'd extend to someone I loved. But love felt too ambitious when I was deep in the trenches of self-criticism. The bar was so low, I would have settled for basic self-respect. Even my inner mean girl deserves a day off here and there, right?

If I could go back to that day on the scale, I wouldn't obsess over the outcome. I would show myself more kindness and shift my focus to the process. The number 273 was a snapshot in time, not a life sentence. I couldn't erase it, and punishing myself certainly wouldn't change it. But I could choose to speak to myself with compassion, and I could remind myself that even though I was struggling, I wasn't a failure, and that I could take things one step at a time. It's like changing your inner soundtrack from depressing ballads to power anthems. It's a deliberate choice to rewrite the narrative.

We all have the power to hit "skip" on the self-sabotaging soundtracks and create our own anthems of resilience. When I finally stopped catastrophizing, I found space for strength, even when things fell off the rails a little.

Muscle Power, Mind Power Tip #8: Trainer Power

L et's talk about 2019, the year my world fell apart.

I was on the cusp of turning 40, an age when I vaguely assumed I would have my act together. Instead, I was separated from my husband, jobless, and doing my best not to trip over my brother's shoes in the apartment we shared. It was a trifecta of setbacks that would have sent even the most stable person spiraling.

But there was still one decision left to make. *The big one.* The life-altering decision you've all been waiting for:

Decision #4: I Hired a Personal Trainer

Okay, I know what you might be thinking: "Oh great, here comes the part where she tells how the personal trainer she hired with her bottomless bank account solved all her problems." You might even be picturing me swanning around my fancy gym, decked out in Lululemon, sipping green juice while I casually wait in line for my pilates class. But before you toss this book aside, thinking it's not for you, let's start by adding some critical context to this decision.

Remember the trifecta of setbacks we just talked about? I had just quit my job with no backup plan. Financially, I wasn't in a position to sign up for a swanky gym membership, much less a personal trainer who costs about as much as an hour with a decent therapist (and *much* more than a really good bottle of wine).

Clearly, my two-step budget plan was:

1. Get fit.
2. Hope for a miracle.

I'd call my decision-making at the time reckless, but I feel like it would be an insult to reckless people everywhere. Objectively, it was a terrible financial strategy. But subjectively, it was a gutsy call made from a place of misplaced and misguided motivation that somehow didn't end in complete financial ruin and, to my astonishment and disbelief, *actually paid off.*

If you have both the desire and the means, I'm living proof that a good trainer and gym access are prudent investments in yourself. While I'd sign on that dotted line again in a recklessly irresponsible, spandex-clad heartbeat, my approach (the one involving no job, a shoestring budget, and a prayer) isn't something I could recommend to anyone in good conscience.

So, *yes*, this story involves a personal trainer (or three!), and *yes*, having access to a gym and trainers is undeniably a *huge* advantage.

But that isn't the whole story.

For every structured session I had with a trainer, I spent countless hours in my own space, often in my pajamas, doing the best I could to figure things out when I didn't have all the answers. I relied on trial and error, learning from my mistakes and gaining real-world experience. What stands out is that the most important lessons, like those about mindset, sustainable habits, and finding what works for you, aren't the exclusive perks of a gym membership and a personal trainer. They apply whether you're in a state-of-the-art facility or making it work on a yoga mat in your living room.

Life has a funny way of hiding its most valuable lessons in the last place you'd ever think to look. Often, it's right in the middle of your most questionable choices. Because I do have a knack for doing everything the hard way, when I finally show up on wisdom's doorstep, I usually arrive looking like I've been dragged backwards through a hedge. My recklessly irresponsible decision to hire a trainer during this especially challenging phase of my life? It stands as Exhibit A. Classic Lisa.

To truly understand how this moment of peak reckless decision-making turned into the choice that changed everything, you need the rest of the origin story. Remember the girl who tossed her belongings out the door and sped away in the middle of the night from the condo she shared with her husband to move into an apartment that can only be described as "Roachella" with her brother?

She's back, and things aren't looking good.

CHAPTER 4

The Insult that Sparked a Revolution

The November night air was crisp as my brother and I pulled up to our new apartment. Under the dim glow of the streetlights, we unloaded our laughably few belongings. We were both running on fumes, and exhaustion was etched into our faces. Reality hit hard as I stepped into my empty bedroom with a garbage bag of clothes in my hand.

I had no bed.

Just four walls and a floor, which ironically mirrored the emptiness of my life.

But my brother, a carpenter with a heart of gold, wasn't about to let his emotionally bruised sister suffer through a sleepless night on the cold, hard floor. With a few scraps of wood and a spare mattress he'd stashed away in his storage locker, he whipped up a makeshift bed. It wasn't much, but it felt like pure love to me. I'll never forget the kindness and understanding he showed me that night.

I tossed some sheets on my new bed, fluffed the pillows, and crashed. The apartment was silent, and I was alone for the first time in a very long time. I thought I would sleep peacefully, but the exhaustion, shame, and fear all converged into a single, overwhelming body and soul ache that night. My brain wouldn't slow down and allow me to rest. Instead, it replayed all the decisions that led me to this point, like my failed marriage, the career I'd burned to the ground, and the broken promises I'd made to myself.

I felt like a colossal failure.

Days bled into one another as I barely left my bed. I lived in a faded Metallica t-shirt and stained sweats that had seen better days. Self-care? Never heard of her. My brother gently nudged me to seek help, to talk to someone, to do anything but continue to wallow in my misery. I'd nod and make promises, but my words were as empty as my motivation. I was stuck, paralyzed by my own inertia.

My brother was patient and understanding. He never judged me, never uttered a harsh word, and was a pillar of strength in the chaos of my life.

That is, until the day he couldn't take it anymore.

After weeks of witnessing my downward spiral, he snapped. Out of love and exasperation, he hurled a verbal grenade my way.

"You're not going to like this, but you need to hear it." He paused, searching for the right words as I braced myself for impact.

"Lisa," he finally said, "you're... *stagnant* and *flaccid*."

I sat there for a full minute with my mouth open processing what he said. Stagnant? That was a blow. But flaccid? *Flaccid*? That hit differently. It stung like a paper cut straight to the soul. I don't care who you are, flaccid is a bad look for anyone.

But he also wasn't wrong. I could have easily used that insult to spiral even further into self-pity. Maybe it was the sheer audacity of the insult, a spark of defiance, or the realization that I refused to be defined by this low point in my life. Whatever it was, it was an odd but surprisingly effective catalyst for change.

Flaccid?

No way. Not me.

Game on.

I dragged myself out of bed, showered, and found something resembling clean clothes in the wreckage of my bedroom. Next, I bit the bullet and booked an appointment with a mental health professional, finally ready to face the burnout head-on. Then, I marched myself straight to the gym.

Yes, the gym.

I know, it seems like a bizarre choice, especially because it had always been a place of self-sabotage, not self-care. I'd always gone too hard, too fast, and quit just as quickly. But in the midst of a life that felt like it was unraveling, the gym was a familiar place. I wanted to hurt, to burn, and to feel the strain in my muscles as a substitute for the ache in my gut. I wanted to punish myself for feeling so lost while simultaneously performing for a world I believed was watching and judging. This had nothing to do with getting healthy. It was about control.

I strode up to the front desk, and before I could give too much thought to what I was about to do, I asked for an entry-level personal training package, plunking down my credit card with a flourish. My dwindling bank account let out a whimper, but I ignored it.

Back in my car, I closed my eyes and slowly exhaled. I was completely drained. I hadn't left my bed, let alone my apartment, in weeks. It took everything I had to walk in the gym and purchase those personal training sessions, forget actually exercising. With the ink still drying on my personal training contract (a startlingly expensive piece of paper, especially considering my poor track record with gym commitment), I made the only promise I felt capable of making at the time. I would show up twice a week, every week, even if all I could manage was dragging my pajama-clad ass through the front doors. No crazy diets, no killer "extra credit" workouts, just that small commitment to myself and my well-being.

This choice wasn't a conscious strategy. It was born from the constraints of my situation. This is how my recklessly irresponsible decision became a genuine commitment to myself, one that would pay dividends in every area of my life.

It forced me to simplify.

My usual "restrict and sacrifice" mentality wouldn't cut it, because my circumstances flat-out wouldn't allow it. The usual overwhelm, the pressure to do everything all at once, and the endless quest for the "perfect" plan? They were immediately off the table because I didn't have the physical or mental resources to manage anything more than the bare minimum, the absolute least I could physically and mentally scrape together and still call it progress.

Going to the gym twice a week might sound like a big commitment to many, but I had no job, no kids, and no responsibilities to speak of, and my days were spent in bed. It was a very reasonable and manageable action I could take. It was my first tiny habit, a small and accidental act of self-care that would become the pebble that started the avalanche.

Though, at the time, it felt less like a life-altering promise with the potential to trigger a natural disaster, and more like the tiniest pebble rolling slowly down a very gentle slope.

The first few weeks were a blur of exhaustion and doubt. It felt like nothing had changed. Aside from the two hours a week I spent at the gym groaning, sweating, and wondering why I signed up for this voluntarily, I continued to spend most of my day in bed. My mental health was a constant battle. I still wasn't sleeping, and the persistent stress of the unknown caused an overwhelming, chaotic clutter of thoughts that I couldn't even begin to organize.

My eating habits weren't exactly worthy of a gold star, either. If the nutrition police existed, I'd be serving a life sentence. Caffeine was my primary food group, with a side of whatever my favorite fast food delivery driver could drop off at my doorstep. I actually got him a Christmas card that year.

But through it all, I stubbornly stuck to my twice-a-week gym commitment.

Slowly, things started to change. I traded in my fast food habit for healthier pre-made meals from the grocery store. I forced myself to drink a glass of water before meals, diluting my dependence on coffee and soda. I knew that my late-night sugar and fat fests were wreaking havoc on my sleep, and as my diet improved and I got more rest, my mood improved. I even started wearing clothes that didn't have holes or stains. I gradually rediscovered the simple pleasures of showering, brushing my hair and teeth, and even putting on a little makeup. Caring for myself and presenting a better version of myself to the world felt good.

To anyone else, my progress would have seemed invisible. But my brother, who'd seen me at my absolute lowest, saw this for what it was.

A resurrection.

A few weeks into my gym routine, he gave me the ultimate compliment. "Lisa," he announced with a grin, "whatever you're doing, keep it up. You're not *flaccid* anymore!" We erupted into a fit of laughter that echoed through our shabby apartment. I felt a lightness I hadn't experienced in months.

As I lay in bed that night, a surprising thought crept into my mind.

"Wait a minute… am I actually… *happy?*"

I closed my eyes with a smile on my face and, for the first time in what felt like forever, drifted off into a peaceful, deep, restful sleep.

Muscle Power, Mind Power Tip #9: "Doing Less" in a "Do More" World

Sitting in my car with my freshly signed personal training contract, I felt a wave of nausea. My inner mean girl, still sipping on a potent cocktail of "no pain, no gain" dogma, sneered, "Is that it?! Two workouts a week? That's never going to be enough to see any kind of progress!" It was so much less than I'd ever forced myself to do before, and it flew directly in the face of a health and fitness world constantly bombarding us with deafening "Do more!" messages demanding relentless, all-or-nothing effort. It's no wonder that the idea of "doing less" feels so counterintuitive.

Beyond the "more is always better" pressure, the entire health and fitness space is a minefield of contradictory advice. One minute, it's "eat more to fuel muscle growth!" then it's "slash calories to see the scale move!" Or the classic, "you need a rigid, follow-every-detail plan!" immediately followed by "but also be super flexible, because life happens!" It's enough to make you want to throw your hands up. We're all drowning in "expert" advice from the latest podcast, guru, or viral reel. It's often conflicting, rarely personalized, and pretty much guaranteed to make you feel like no matter what you choose, you're inevitably doing it wrong.

We get so busy trying to decipher everyone else's "shoulds" and "must dos" that we forget or even ignore the incredibly intelligent feedback system we were born with: Our own bodies. We have the most sophisticated, intuitive GPS imaginable right inside us,

81

but we've muted its calm, wise voice to listen to a cacophony of backseat drivers all shouting conflicting directions at the top of their lungs instead.

The exciting (and often wildly frustrating) truth about transformation is that you are both the scientist *and* the guinea pig in your own personal laboratory. The objective of your experiment isn't to find the one set of external rules that works for everyone, it's to chart your own path. It's a gentle, practical process of small-scale trial and pint-sized error, enabled by two non-negotiable mindset shifts:

1. Give yourself permission to "do less" in a "do more" world.
2. Reframe failure as learning to build self-knowledge.

This is where BJ Fogg's idea of starting ridiculously small, which we touched on earlier, comes into play. Maybe your "tiny food experiment" was to add kale to your dinners, only to discover that it tastes like something even your compost bin would politely decline. You didn't "blow your diet" when you trashed the kale and ate something you actually enjoyed, you gathered helpful intel. So tomorrow, you try eating broccoli instead. Perhaps your plan to hit the gym for a pre-dawn workout was hijacked by your comfy bed and the snooze button. You're not "lazy," but maybe quick walks after meals become your new, more realistic experiment. They're easy pivots with no drama, and data points guiding you to what clicks.

We're fed a steady diet of unrealistic, unsustainable messages, yet we rarely question them. When we inevitably fall short, instead of challenging the narrative, we internalize the failure by believing that we're the problem. This leads us down the short path toward crushing ourselves under the weight of "I just didn't try hard enough."

Given my propensity for making things much harder than they need to be, I'm practically a credentialed expert in the art of "oops." I thought blowing up my life would be my rock bottom, but my subsequent "stagnant and flaccid" era took it a giant leap further. In retrospect, this wasn't a surprise. That period was the entirely predictable result of an embarrassingly long time spent diligently accumulating a generous pile of illuminating failures. I borrowed the term from NASA engineers who use it to explain the process of scrutinizing what goes wrong to learn and improve. I figured if it's good enough for rocket scientists, it's good enough for me! The most illuminating part was realizing the common denominator was my unwavering commitment to doing things the hard way.

Failure is only an effective teacher if you're internalizing the lessons. Otherwise, it's just an unfortunate event. The cycle of falling, dusting myself off, and mustering the audacity to try again with a revised approach is what finally started to chip away at what I'd call my rather spectacular level of "self-ignorance". While "lack of self-awareness" is the more widely accepted term, it feels like it falls short of the gold-standard of "self-cluelessness" I was rocking at the time. It was by internalizing the insights from each of those stumbles that I started to build genuine self-knowledge.

It wasn't until that day, sitting in my car after spending a pile of money I knew I didn't have, that I paused to consider if a different, let alone gentler, approach might work better for me. That thought didn't surface because I believed it was the right thing for me at the time, but because I didn't have the strength to do anything else. Leave it to me to find the right path not through some grand epiphany or moment of clarity, but by simply being too tired to keep going down the wrong one.

What looks like failure is often just the universe handing you illuminating data to help clarify your direction. When you see it that way, the shame evaporates. By understanding that each misstep has the potential to reveal something important, I slowly replaced my "self-ignorance" with self-knowledge.

When you have the confidence to try and fail repeatedly while still believing with all your heart that the next attempt will change everything, sustainable progress doesn't just become possible, it becomes practically inevitable.

CHAPTER 5

The Unexpected Gifts of Weightlifting – A Love Letter to Myself

How did I go from feeling overwhelmed and stuck to finding that glimmer of happiness, even with all the challenges I was facing? Let's go back to late 2019, to the day I walked into the gym for my first personal training session, a day that would change everything.

I arrived at the gym and stood at the foot of the grand, winding staircase leading to the workout floor. For someone whose exercise routine mainly consisted of sporadic elliptical sessions and brisk walks to the fridge, it may as well have been Mount Everest. As I faced those steps, they held more fear than promise.

If you're nervous about making a change and unsure of where to start, I get it. If you had told the version of me standing at the bottom of the stairs that day, the girl who could barely muster the energy to swap pajamas for a sports bra, that the gym would eventually become a place where she felt truly at home in her own skin, she would have laughed in your face.

Or maybe burst into tears. It was a volatile time.

My brother's cruel (but also hilariously accurate) words echoed in my ears as I climbed. *Stagnant* and *flaccid*. "Stagnant and Flaccid Lisa" was the version of me I was determined to leave behind. She would have turned back and let her expensive personal training contract become another donation to the gym.

But I knew I couldn't keep running away from my problems. I needed to confront my fears head-on. I had to prove to myself, and to "Stagnant and Flaccid Lisa," that I was capable of more.

Anxiety washed over me as I climbed. It felt like every eye in the gym was on me, judging my labored breathing and my less-than-athletic gym outfit. The weight room came into view, a foreign place filled with intimidating machines and athletic-looking people. I felt like a lost tourist in a place I didn't belong.

If I could travel back in time and talk to that terrified woman on the stairs, this is what I'd say:

"Lisa, keep walking up those stairs because there is so much unexpected joy waiting for you.

The confidence you're about to build in the gym will spill over into every area of your life, transforming your relationships and deepening your connections with the people you love. You'll stop just existing, sitting on the couch, waiting for another day to pass you by. You'll transform into someone who shows up fully and embraces adventures big and small. You'll become the friend your loved ones can count on, and the daughter and sister who brings laughter and light to your family.

It's going to change your career, too. Instead of hiding in the comfort of mediocrity, you'll work hard and take chances. That initiative will put you in the path of a former boss, someone you respect deeply, and who recognizes your potential. She'll believe in you, giving you a chance to shine. You'll work tirelessly to earn the confidence she placed in you, proving her right time and time again. With each accomplishment, you'll build a career that once seemed out of reach, a career you didn't think was possible for someone like you.

It will also change your love life in ways you can't even imagine. You'll realize there's more out there than you ever dreamed of, including the most incredible man you've ever known. He'll love the real you, not the one you've been hiding behind your insecurities, and he'll inspire, challenge, and support you like no one has before.

But this love isn't going to come in the package you expect.

He's going to be shorter than you!

I know his height is a dealbreaker for you now, which is a reflection of your insecurities about your size. But strength training will give you the courage and confidence to embrace happiness, no matter what shape it takes. You'll build an incredible life with your "Short King," filled with love, laughter, and adventures. And the height difference that seems like such a big deal today? It'll become a playful inside joke between two people deeply in love.

The mental makeover will be the unexpected bonus you didn't realize you needed. But I know you didn't walk through the gym doors today for a therapy session.

You want to see results.

You want to build a body you love that makes you feel beautiful, strong, and confident. And let me tell you, the physical changes will blow you away. When you finally abandon your old "restrict and sacrifice" mentality and start nourishing your body and challenging yourself in the gym, you'll build a physique that's not just strong and healthy, but downright stunning. Those sculpted shoulders you've always dreamed of? They're coming. That narrow waist that complements your curvy hips and thighs? Absolutely.

Adding muscle won't just give you the hourglass figure you've always wanted, it'll also boost your metabolism. Right now, you feel like every bite shows up on your hips. Resistance training will change that. You'll become the envy of your friends, effortlessly enjoying a glass of wine and dessert without a second thought. You'll understand that occasional treats won't derail your progress because you've built a solid foundation of healthy habits, and the occasional delicious dessert will fuel an amazing workout the next day.

And speaking of amazing workouts, get ready to fall head over heels for the feeling of strength. It's a feeling that's hard to articulate, but once you've felt it, you'll never forget it. Ripping a heavy weight off the floor isn't just a physical act, it's an act of power that makes everything else in your life feel a little easier. Building physical strength is an emotional journey as much as a physical one, and it will give you a kind of resilience that changes how you see yourself and the world.

There's one last thing I need to tell you.

I wish I didn't have to because I would do anything to spare you the heartache, but it's a crucial part of your story.

Your mom, the strongest, most vibrant woman you know—the one who never misses her daily walks with her adorable dog Teddy, her aquafit classes, or her weekly golf games with the girls—will be diagnosed with breast cancer. It's a cruel twist of fate and an unimaginable blow that will hit you hard. You won't be able to reconcile how this can happen to someone so full of life and love.

In true mom fashion, she'll put on a brave face to shield you from her fear. But the cancer treatments will take their toll, relentlessly chipping away at her energy and vitality. Everyday tasks will become a struggle, and it will break your heart to witness her fight and hold her hand as she grapples with a vulnerability she's never allowed herself to show.

When it comes to hardships like illness or injury, it's not a matter of if it happens, but when. That's when the power of physical strength becomes undeniably crucial. Through your mom's experience, you'll come to understand, perhaps in a way you can't fully grasp now, the true value of resistance training and building muscle. It's about living a vibrant, independent, and healthy life well into your later years with the strength and resilience to persevere, no matter what life throws your way.

Through the pain and uncertainty, there will be hope. Your mom's active lifestyle will equip her to face her cancer treatments with the spirit of a survivor. She'll persevere with the tenacity of a champion, bouncing back stronger and more determined than ever before. She'll also make positive lifestyle changes, losing more than 60 pounds herself, motivated by her diagnosis but inspired by you.

I'm telling you this because I need you to know that your journey will be hard, and there will be moments when you want to give up.

Please don't.

In the end, you'll look back and smile, knowing the beautiful life in store for you.

So keep walking up those stairs, Lisa. This health, this happiness, this physical and mental strength and resilience, it's all yours for the taking."

My love affair with resistance training didn't start with a burning passion for barbells or a deep understanding of fitness. It began with a single, hesitant step up those intimidating stairs. That's why my passion for weightlifting runs deep, and why I can't help but share its benefits with anyone with the patience to listen. I've witnessed firsthand the power it holds to transform bodies and lives.

No matter where you are on your journey, you deserve to experience that same power. You deserve to live and age with vitality, strength, and purpose.

Muscle Power, Mind Power Tip #10:
10 Downsides of Dodging Dumbbells

If the last section didn't make it abundantly clear, I'll say it out loud here.

I'm biased when it comes to weight training.

It was so transformative for me that I can be borderline evangelical about it. I'm not afraid to shout its benefits from the rooftops (or, you know, write a whole book about it!). And given that the book has *"Muscle Power"* right in the title, I'd be willing to bet that you're expecting to find at least a decent chunk dedicated to the power of lifting weights.

And you'd be right.

While it's absolutely true that any movement you enjoy and can stick with consistently is foundational, there's a special kind of power reserved for resistance training. If you want to build serious real-world strength, functional capability, and the kind of long-term resilience that'll help you dodge some genuinely unpleasant potential health issues down the road, then we *really* need to focus the conversation on building muscle.

Sometimes, knowing what you don't want is a lot more motivating than knowing what you do. So, forget what we stand to gain for a second, and let's talk about the downsides. I've come up with a list of ten rather compelling (and not-so-glamorous) negative consequences of skipping the weights. I'm not expecting all of these "don'ts" to hit home for you. But sometimes, it just takes one specific "Oof, I really don't want that!" realization for things to click into place.

1. Weaker Bones

I don't want a little stumble to turn into a full-blown fracture.

As we age, our bones naturally become a bit more fragile. (Thanks, hormones!) However, weight-bearing exercises stimulate bone growth and help maintain density. As a Canadian girl who's lived through her fair share of cold winters, you can trust me when I say that a tumble on the ice is much less scary when you have a solid foundation.

2. Decreased Muscle Mass

I don't want to utter the words, "I've fallen, and I can't get up."

Age-related muscle loss (sarcopenia) is a natural part of aging. But strength training can help you build and maintain muscle mass, slowing down or even reversing those effects. A little extra muscle might mean the difference between lying on your back, limbs flailing like an overturned turtle, and the ability to flip yourself over and get back up.

3. Decreased Mobility, Balance, and Coordination

I don't want my body to feel like a restriction, holding me back from experiences.

Training opens up a world of possibilities for me to live life to the fullest. This means adventures with my future grandkids and eventually embarrassing them with my killer 90s dance moves at their weddings. You can't successfully execute the "worm" with good form at 85 years old if you don't have good mobility, balance, and coordination!

4. Slower Metabolism

I don't want my body's metabolic "thermostat" to feel permanently stuck on "low."

A strong metabolism means more flexibility and less food-related anxiety. Muscle tissue is more metabolically active than fat, which means it burns more calories even at rest. So, the more muscle you have, the easier it is to maintain a healthy weight. This lets you occasionally indulge in "sometimes" foods without derailing your goals.

5. Lousy Mood

I don't want "generally grumpy," "easily frazzled," or "chronically unenthusiastic" to be my baseline personality.

Weight training acts as a natural mood booster by triggering the release of endorphins, the feel-good chemicals in your brain. It's also an incredibly effective way to channel stress, anxiety, or even a bad mood into something positive and productive.

6. Decreased Energy

I don't want to feel like I'm running on fumes, struggling to get through even basic daily tasks.

Weightlifting naturally enhances energy levels by increasing cardiovascular health, improving blood flow, and boosting the function of the mitochondria in your cells (where the energy from food is converted into usable form for your body).

7. Increased Risk of Chronic Diseases

I don't want my daily life to become a schedule of medications and doctor visits for problems that were largely preventable.

Strength training is like an investment in a long, vibrant future. It can help reduce the risk of chronic diseases like heart disease, Type 2 diabetes, and even some types of cancer. It achieves this by improving cardiovascular health, supporting a healthy body composition, and promoting better blood sugar control and hormonal balance.

8. Decreased Insulin Sensitivity and Blood Sugar Regulation

I don't want the simple joy of occasionally eating cheesecake to feel like a forbidden pleasure.

As we age, our bodies can become less efficient at processing sugar. Resistance training can help improve insulin sensitivity, which means your body can use glucose for energy more effectively. Muscles act as a primary storage site for glucose, so building muscle mass helps pull excess sugars from your bloodstream, contributing to more stable blood sugar levels. This leads to improved energy levels throughout the day. It also reduces your risk of developing Type 2 diabetes and other metabolic disorders.

9. Insomnia

I don't want to rely on pharmaceuticals for a good night's rest.

Resistance training can significantly improve sleep quality by reducing stress hormones, regulating circadian rhythms, and tiring you out (in a good way!). This leaves you feeling refreshed and energized in the morning, with a clearer head and a brighter mood.

10. Low Confidence

I don't want my potential to go unrealized because I didn't have the confidence to step up and own it.

While I expected to gain physical strength in the weight room, I wasn't prepared for the internal overhaul that accompanied it. Weightlifting taught me resilience, discipline, and the power of pushing past my perceived limits. It gave me the confidence to embrace challenges in the gym and all areas of my life. I learned that I was capable of more than I ever thought possible. That realization fundamentally changed how I approached obstacles and pursued my goals.

Strength training transformed my body, mind, and entire outlook on life. It can do the same for you, no matter who you are, your age, your life stage, or your physical ability.

Muscle Power, Mind Power Tip #11:
The Gym is a Happy, Safe Place

The gym might be the last place you want to spend your time. There are countless ways to move your body and challenge your muscles, and you don't need a gym membership to do it. The gym is just one option, and it's definitely not for everyone. If you have no desire to set foot in a gym, feel free to skip ahead.

I promise I won't be offended!

But let's say I piqued your interest with my list of *"10 Big Don'ts,"* and now, you're gym-curious. Or maybe you've always wanted to try weightlifting, but haven't quite mustered the courage to walk through those intimidating doors. This section is for you. I'm here to share my experience and hopefully dispel some myths, fears, and "gymtimidation" that might hold you back.

1. Everyone at the gym already looks like a fitness model.

This is as true as saying everyone who cooks is a Michelin-star chef.

The gym is full of perfectly imperfect people of all ages, shapes, sizes, and fitness levels who are there to learn, grow, and challenge themselves. Sure, you'll catch the occasional six-pack. But you're far more likely to see folks just trying to get a little stronger, healthier, and maybe feel more comfortable in their skin. We've all got jiggly bits, cellulite, messy hair, and sweat stains, but we've

THE UNEXPECTED GIFTS OF WEIGHTLIFTING – A LOVE LETTER TO MYSELF

also got the determination to keep showing up. That's the real beauty of the gym. It's a celebration of effort, not perfection.

So, don't let comparison steal your joy, motivation, or your chance to become the best version of yourself.

2. Everyone is watching and judging your every move.

Have you ever noticed how many people at the gym wear headphones? It's not just for the music. Headphones create a personal space, a little bubble of focus where you can "lock in" to your workout without distractions. Most people at the gym are in their own world, tuned into their goals and playlists, and tuned out of their surroundings.

Unless you're doing something truly extraordinary or unusual, you're probably blending right in. We've all been beginners, struggling with a new exercise or feeling self-conscious. That shared experience triggers empathy, not judgment.

3. You need a PhD in Exercise Science to walk through the door.

It's confession time.

When I first started, I thought a "lat pulldown" was a type of window shade and that a "skull crusher" belonged in a horror movie. Thankfully, it's just a tricep exercise!

The gym can seem like it has its own language and a million complicated machines. But there are simple ways to get comfortable. Start with the machines, because they often have diagrams showing how to use them, and they're generally safer for beginners than other options. Take a few minutes to watch what other people are doing, or ask a staff member for help. Most gyms offer an orientation session, so take advantage of it! It's a great way to learn the layout, familiarize yourself with the equipment, and ask any questions.

You'll learn as you go, and before you know it, you'll be busting out "good mornings" (which are so much more than just a polite greeting—they're a deceptively tough exercise for your glutes and hamstrings) with the skill and precision of a seasoned pro.

4. There are too many options, and you don't know where to start.

The sheer variety at the gym can be overwhelming at first. There's your cardio bunnies, your weightlifting warriors, and let's not forget your group fitness fanatics. It's a lot to take in. Try to see it as an opportunity to experiment and find what you genuinely enjoy. Start with something small, like a brisk walk on the treadmill or a few basic weight machines.

Once you feel more comfortable, explore other options and see where they lead. Maybe you'll discover a love for spin classes or find your inner peace in yoga. And if you accidentally try something that's not your style (I'm looking at you, Zumba!), it's no big deal because there's plenty more to choose from. Many gyms offer a wide range of group fitness classes, which can be a fun and social way to try new things.

5. You're worried about getting hurt.

It's natural to worry about injury, especially when you're starting something new. But as a woman who out-lifted her back problems, I can tell you that you're much more likely to pull something sneezing or putting on your socks than you are to get injured in the gym. The key is to start slowly, listen to your body, learn proper form, and be patient with yourself.

You're not just working out, you're learning a new skill.

6. You don't have time to go to the gym regularly.

Between work, family, social life, and trying to squeeze in those elusive 7-9 hours of sleep, who has time for hours at the gym? The idea that a workout needs to be a marathon session to be effective is a lie.

20-30 minutes a couple of times a week will add up over time. It's about consistency, not duration. You don't need to read an entire book in one sitting to get something out of it, right?

What's even better about this trick is that the little victory you feel after completing a short workout gives your brain an associated mini-boost, making you *want* to find other small ways to move throughout the day.

7. You're afraid of breaking an unwritten gym rule and embarrassing yourself.

Ah, the dreaded "gym etiquette." There are some unspoken rules, but they mostly boil down to courtesy and respect. Here's the lowdown:

Do: Wipe down your equipment. Seriously, no one wants your sweat.

Don't: Camp out on a machine scrolling through your social media feed. You paid the same price of admission as everyone else, so be respectful of others waiting to use the equipment. A little self-awareness goes a long way!

Do: Be mindful of personal space. If 20 treadmills are free, don't get on the one next to someone else. But if it's busy, everything is fair game!

Don't: Grunt excessively loud. While a little "uuugh!" on your last rep is understandable (and might even earn you a nod of solidarity for pushing through the burn), drowning out everyone else's music with your sound effects is a no-go.

Do: Use hand signals to communicate. Pointing down at a machine with a questioning look is gym-speak for "Are you using this?" Holding up one, two, and then three fingers means, "How many sets do you have left? I want to use this after you."

Don't: Try to strike up a conversation with someone who's clearly in the zone (headphones on, "locked in" to their workout). That said, a friendly smile and a head nod to acknowledge someone are always welcome. It's a simple way of saying, "Enjoy your workout!"

It's mostly common sense. And if you accidentally break a rule, relax. It happens. Laugh it off, learn from it, and move on. The gym police aren't going to kick you out for a minor slip-up.

Believe it or not, the gym can be a surprisingly happy and safe space. It's a place where people from all walks of life come together, united by the shared mission of personal growth. We may be at different stages in our journeys, but we all understand the sweat and the struggle. This shared experience creates a unique camaraderie. A nod between sets or an exhausted smile after a challenging class is all it takes to know we're all in this together.

And because we're all in it together, don't hesitate to ask for help. As a now-experienced gym-goer, I'm genuinely thrilled when a newbie approaches me. It's a chance to share what I've learned and welcome someone new into the fold.

If "gymtimidation" has been your barrier, take a deep breath, put on your favorite workout gear, and head to the gym. You might be surprised at what you find there.

CHAPTER 6

Trainer #1 – Torching Calories

This is the part where I get into some of my most illuminating failures, the most embarrassing, humbling moments from the early days of my fitness journey. It's your backstage pass to the messy, imperfect, and often hilarious process of transformation. I hope you'll see through the lens of my experience that you don't need to have it all figured out before you take your first steps.

The goal is to make mistakes and learn as you go.

I've had the pleasure and privilege of working with three amazing personal trainers throughout my journey. Each one brought their unique personality and expertise to the table, shaping my story in different ways. To keep things simple, I'll refer to them as Trainer #1, #2, and #3. Don't get me wrong; this isn't to downplay how much they mean to me or their role in my transformation. They all know that I'm deeply grateful for everything they taught me. But for the sake of storytelling, let's just go with the numbers.

Without further ado, allow me to introduce you to Trainer #1.

After what felt like an eternity (or at least a chapter or two!) climbing that winding staircase, I finally reached the top, slightly out of breath but determined. Stepping onto the gym floor, I was a bundle of nerves but ready to face whatever Trainer #1 had in store.

I was taking my first wobbly steps toward a new me, and I wasn't looking back.

Trainer #1 had an infectious energy, and his warm smile instantly put me at ease in this intimidating new environment. Our initial consultation felt a bit like a fitness confessional. I revealed the truth about my exercise history (or, more accurately, lack thereof), confessed my most ambitious fitness desires, and shared a few dietary sins. With nothing to lose, I laid it all out there. I explained that I wanted to lose weight and was ready to do whatever it took. He confidently assured me that we'd conquer those goals together.

After that first session, I felt the tiniest twinge of hope. I dared to allow myself to consider that maybe, *just maybe*, I could actually pull this off.

I loved Trainer #1 because he listened to what I asked for and then cranked it up to eleven. He designed calorie-torching workouts that were a relentless, grueling test of my limits. Given my extensive background in self-inflicted elliptical misery, I figured this was just the price of admission for a successful fitness routine. I'd leave each session depleted, drenched in sweat, and sometimes even in tears.

One session in particular stands out in my memory.

We were nearing the end of an especially brutal workout when Trainer #1 instructed me to do some weighted step-ups. As a newbie lifter, it was a big ask. Dutifully, I picked up my weights and got to work.

But the workout had been tough, and I was out of gas. Only a few reps in, my heart started hammering against my ribs, my muscles were screaming in agony, and my legs felt like they were about to give out altogether. My body was waving the white flag of surrender. Still, stubbornness and a desperate need to prove myself took over. I pushed through, despite my blurry vision and a wave of nausea. The thought of seeing the disappointment in Trainer #1's eyes, of him thinking I was weak or incapable, was all I needed to keep going despite my obvious physical distress.

It's clear to me now that my motivation wasn't exactly rooted in the healthiest of places, but at the time, it was the only thing keeping me moving.

I gritted my teeth, ignoring the rising panic in my chest. Suddenly, my world narrowed, and my body felt like it was about to shut down altogether. My breathing became rapid and shallow. Each gasp was a desperate plea for oxygen. Mortified, I realized I was hyperventilating in front of a gym full of strangers. It was the worst-case scenario and the ultimate gym-fail nightmare came to life.

Trainer #1 remained calm, the picture of professionalism, and quickly came to my side. Unfazed by my dramatic display of gasping and wheezing, he quietly guided me through breathing exercises until I regained control. With shaky legs and an even shakier resolve, I wiped away the tears and picked up my weights. Collapsing in a puddle of shame on the gym floor seemed like a fate far worse than pushing through the discomfort of finishing my set.

But that didn't stop me from having a full-on meltdown in the bathroom stall immediately after my workout. This wasn't a pretty cry where a few stray tears stream down your otherwise perfect face. It was the kind of ugly cry that (ironically) left me gasping for air between sobs.

With snot leaking down my face, I felt defeated. How could I face Trainer #1 again after he'd witnessed my pathetic display of weakness and vulnerability?

Back home in the familiar safety of my bed, sporting my favorite old Metallica t-shirt and worn-in sweatpants, I thought about never going back. The workout wasn't just hard, it felt like proof that I was out of my depth. Deep in the feeling of embarrassment, I pictured Trainer #1 chuckling with his colleagues about the "dramatic newbie" who was "completely incapable" and a certified "lost cause."

After feeling so raw and exposed, the desire to hide under the covers and fade away was impossible to ignore. So I didn't. I leaned into it. Retreating felt like a necessary act of self-care, giving me time to feel my feelings and process what had happened.

So, I gave the floor to my inner mean girl, and allowed her to have her moment. She smugly stepped into the spotlight, and launched into her typical narrative.

"You're not cut out for this," she began, stifling a bored yawn. "This new path isn't you. Your old routine of self-inflicted elliptical misery is where you belong." Then came the dagger. "Some people just aren't built for success, and you're one of them. It's not a big deal. Just go back to what's comfortable and give up." She added the final blow under her breath, just loud enough for me to hear, "You always do eventually." Quitting was the path of least resistance, and easy had a powerful appeal right then.

But lying there, stewing in those negative thoughts, I realized that hiding didn't fix anything. I needed to actively confront the defeatist story she was peddling, and for the first time, I actually felt equipped to do it. Weeks of determined consistency had opened up a new file in my mental cabinet labeled "Evidence I'm Not a Complete Failure," and it was getting thicker by the day. Armed with the ammunition I needed, the cross-examination began.

My inner mean girl took the stand, confident in her case. She presented her evidence, using my own thoughts against me: I was a "dramatic newbie," "completely incapable," and a "lost cause."

But this time, I was ready to fight back.

"You call me a dramatic newbie?" I asked her. "Didn't I suffer legitimate physical and mental distress on the gym floor that day?"

"You say I'm completely incapable?" I looked her dead in the eye. "Weren't all my efforts before this evidence that I was capable?"

Finally, I asked the question that mattered most: "Am I a lost cause? Am I really going to accept that as truth based on one negative experience? One vulnerable moment didn't erase weeks of effort, did it? And even if everyone was secretly laughing at me, was their opinion worth sacrificing my goals?"

Keeping my promise felt bigger than the fear. I didn't want "Stagnant and Flaccid Lisa" to be my defining label. I was determined to prove to myself (and, let's be honest, to Trainer #1) that I could face adversity.

Despite the humiliating and humbling blow to my ego and pride, I went back.

Walking into the gym for my next session, I braced myself for the awkward pity, the poorly concealed smirks from the other trainers, and maybe even an outright "So, try not to hyperventilate today, huh?" from Trainer #1. I was so nervous that I felt physically ill.

Despite the catastrophe playing out in my head, Trainer #1 never made me feel judged or incapable. In fact, he pushed me just as hard as before, maybe even harder. His mantra of "Last set, best set!" encouraged me to dig deep, find reserves of strength I never knew I had, and persevere. I wasn't setting any records and wasn't suddenly fearless, but I was *there*, facing the discomfort head-on.

At the end of the workout, earning Trainer #1's encouragement and signature fist bump felt like proof that showing up, even when I was scared, was the most important rep I could do.

In those first few months, I had two main cheerleaders: Trainer #1, of course, and surprisingly, the scale. I lost nearly 60 pounds, bringing me tantalizingly close to a weight I hadn't seen in decades. The elusive 100s finally seemed within reach. It was exhilarating, at least until I faced the mirror. Somehow, my reflection didn't seem to align with that number. I looked a little smaller, sure. But did I look fitter? More capable? Stronger?

Not really.

It was confusing and, honestly, pretty demoralizing. My body was shrinking but not reshaping in the way I'd expected. The visual wasn't keeping pace with the number. My reflection wasn't on the same journey. It was stubbornly lagging behind, stuck in a perpetual state of "before."

But why? I was doing *everything* right, wasn't I?

And, true to form for pretty much anything involving us complicated humans (especially in the complex world of health and fitness), the answer wasn't simple. It was once again, *"Yes... but also, most definitely, no."*

Alongside all the sweat and effort, there were some crucial missteps.

I realize how lucky I was that Trainer #1 was a bit of an evil genius. He gave me exactly what I *thought* I wanted—workouts that felt like a calorie-torching inferno. He was smart enough to know I would walk if he didn't meet me where I was, still deep in my "if it ain't the elliptical, it ain't happening" era.

But here's the catch he understood. When you combine intense calorie-burning workouts with insufficient fuel (especially protein), your body doesn't just burn fat, it also starts sacrificing precious muscle tissue. That's often the culprit behind the "smaller-but-not-fitter" look. Muscle is dense and provides shape, and losing it along with fat can leave you looking less defined or even "soft" despite the lower number on the scale.

That's why Trainer #1 also subtly and persistently tried to steer me toward what I truly *needed*. Let's break it down.

Trainer #1 was relentless in his emphasis on proper nutrition. He stressed the importance of eating enough to support my workouts and overall energy levels while maintaining a modest calorie deficit for continued fat loss. He was particularly adamant about consuming adequate protein for building muscle and recovery.

For me, the idea of adding more protein to my diet conjured up images of bodybuilders chugging protein shakes while bench pressing at the gym. I was there to torch calories, not to build my biceps, so I couldn't help it when my eyes glazed over as he spoke. Patiently, he tried to convince me that protein was about so much more than bulging biceps, emphasizing that maintaining muscle mass was crucial for a healthy metabolism, which would, in turn, support my fat loss goals.

I smiled and nodded as I consistently ignored his good advice, stuck in the old "restrict and sacrifice" mindset. My logic was undeniably flawed when it came to nutrition. If a little restriction is good, *more* must be better, right? Even though I incorporated a pathetic sliver of chicken here and a dollop of Greek yogurt there (which, in hindsight, was still a big win!), it wasn't enough to mitigate the negative impacts of under-eating protein, in particular.

Trainer #1 also managed to pry me away from the elliptical for long enough to teach me the fundamentals of lifting. He helped me improve my mobility so I could lift with proper form, which he explained was crucial for preventing injuries and maximizing muscle activation. He taught me how to properly brace my core to protect my back and create a stable base for my lifts. And, he introduced me to progressive overload, explaining that I needed to continually challenge my muscles by gradually increasing the weight, reps, or sets over time so that my body would adapt and grow stronger.

Thanks to his expertise, my muscle loss wasn't as drastic as it could have been. He expertly blended the strength training my body needed with the calorie-torching I craved. His approach not only kept me engaged and at the gym twice a week, but it prevented me from getting in my own way and completely sabotaging my progress.

Blinded by the lower number on the scale and the allure of a sub-200-pound body, in true Lisa fashion, I doubled down on my effort. I asked Trainer #1 to ramp up our sessions from two to three times a week. Fewer calories, more sweat, an even smaller number on the scale—I was convinced this approach was the fast track to my dream physique.

But life rarely follows a perfectly scripted fitness transformation story.

As I mentally prepared for a more intense routine, disaster struck. Trainer #1 got injured, sidelining him for an agonizingly long six months, maybe longer.

My immediate reaction was sheer panic. There was no way I could move forward without him. Looking back, I cringe at how deeply I distrusted my ability to push myself. In my mind, he was behind the wheel while I was along for the ride. I conveniently forgot that I was the one dragging myself to the gym twice a week, doing the work, and making better food choices.

Because of that misplaced dependence, the idea of starting over with someone new wasn't just overwhelming, it felt downright absurd. I stubbornly refused to entertain the idea that anyone else could fill Trainer #1's shoes. The gym manager's repeated assurance that a new trainer could seamlessly take over for Trainer #1 was met with a healthy dose of skepticism and, let's be honest, melodrama. How could anyone replace the person who had been so instrumental in my transformation?

But with a signed contract and a stack of unused personal training sessions, I was out of options. With a heavy heart, I reluctantly agreed to meet with Trainer #2, convinced it would be a waste of my time.

Trainer #1's unexpected and unceremonious exit marked a bittersweet end to a pivotal chapter in my life. He was there with me from the beginning, patiently teaching me the basics and laying the groundwork for my future success. And to think I judged him right out of the gate by consistently ignoring his advice. It was shortsighted foolishness that could have ended my journey before it even started. Thankfully, Trainer #1's expertise and patience outweighed my stubbornness and resistance to change. He saw the bigger picture when I was chasing quick fixes, pushed me when I needed it most, held me accountable when all

I wanted to do was quit, and guided me toward a success I hadn't quite allowed myself to imagine.

I'll always be grateful to Trainer #1 for being the mentor I never knew I needed and now can't imagine my life without.

Ready or not, I had to turn the page. It was time to embrace a new trainer and a whole new perspective on what it meant to transform my body and my life.

Muscle Power, Mind Power Tip #12: I'm No Mind Reader, But I Am Pretty Good at Overthinking

Let's rewind to that less-than-glamorous moment when I was hyperventilating on the gym floor. It felt like the ultimate public humiliation that makes you want to crawl under a treadmill and never come out.

Hiding in the bathroom, tears streaming down my face, I was spiraling. "How can I ever show my face here again?" I thought, convinced everyone was judging me, secretly laughing at my very public meltdown.

As if on cue, my inner mean girl started to play a cruel game of "Guess What Your Trainer Thinks of You!" and the options she came up with weren't exactly flattering.

> "She's *way* too out of shape."
> "She's a hopeless case."
> "She's wasting my time."
> "*Thank God* she's paying me to be here."

This is a classic example of "mind reading." It's a cognitive distortion in which you assume you know what others are thinking, usually something negative about yourself, without any evidence. In that moment, it felt like my inner mean girl had taken over the broadcast system in my brain, projecting all my worst fears and insecurities onto the people around me.

It's funny (in a not-so-funny way) how our brains can work against us in those vulnerable moments. When we feel exposed or insecure, we subconsciously seek information confirming our negative self-perceptions. This is why we tend to jump to negative mind reading conclusions. Our brains are primed to interpret ambiguous social cues as critical or judgmental because they align with the awful things our inner mean girl is already telling us. The paradox is that in those spiraling moments, we're operating purely on assumption, building elaborate narratives without a single concrete fact to support them.

So, in those moments of self-doubt and anxiety, I remind myself that I can't actually read minds, no matter how convincing my inner mean girl sounds. Instead of immediately leaping to that catastrophic worst-case scenario my brain loves to invent, I try to consciously consider other, more neutral possibilities. Or, even better, I've learned to take the (often scary) step of actually talking to the person I'm worried about. More often than not, a simple, direct conversation is enough to deflate those overblown fears and bring me back to reality.

Swallowing my pride and stepping back onto the gym floor after *The Great Hyperventilation Incident* was a defining moment. The world didn't end, and Trainer #1 was far more supportive and understanding than my anxious mind had led me to believe. It was a powerful lesson in not letting my insecurities dictate my actions.

So, the next time your brain starts spinning those "everyone must think…" scenarios, hit the mental pause button. Remember, those thoughts aren't undeniable truths beamed directly from other people's minds. Reality has a funny way of being less dramatic and surprisingly kinder than the horror stories we invent in our heads. And even if someone *is* judging you, their opinion doesn't define your worth or your potential. Ultimately, the only voice that gets a permanent microphone in your head is your own.

You're stronger than your fears and more capable than you think. Progress often lies just beyond the barriers we create in our own minds. And boy, did I ever have a big barrier in my mind as I contemplated returning to the gym to meet Trainer #2 after learning of Trainer #1's injury.

CHAPTER 7

Trainer #2 (Part 1) – An Unexpected Friendship (and Unexpected Gains)

It's early 2020, only a few short days after receiving that dreaded phone call about Trainer #1's injury. I barely had time to process my grief before I was once again huffing and puffing up that infamous, winding staircase at my gym—the one with its own character arc in my story. This time, it wasn't just the physical exertion that made the climb tough. It was the ache of disappointment, the bitter taste of interrupted progress, and the anxiety of facing this journey without Trainer #1 weighing me down.

My loyalty to Trainer #1 was absolute, and my heart just wasn't in starting over, especially with a stranger, so I went into my meeting with Trainer #2 already convinced it wouldn't work.

Trainer #2 was pleasant enough as he introduced himself and shook my hand. My first reaction wasn't curiosity, but critical comparison. Trainer #1's radiant energy was gone, replaced by an intimidatingly huge brick wall with shoulders. I genuinely wondered if he had to turn sideways to fit through the gym doors. My cynicism kicked into high gear, and my inner mean girl didn't waste the opportunity.

"Trainer #2 won't understand your goals at all," she interjected, oozing with fake concern. "He probably eats raw eggs for breakfast and thinks anything less than a two-hour-long workout is slacking off."

I dismissed him immediately based entirely on the unrelatable "gym bro" label I slapped on him. Clearly, I hadn't learned a thing about not judging people from my experience with Trainer #1. It wasn't a good look for me.

Sadly, I wasn't winning any Miss Congeniality awards that day, either. As we sat together, I slumped down in my chair and rolled my eyes as he initiated a second round of "So, tell me about your health and fitness goals…" It felt like I was stuck in a terrible, low-budget sequel to a movie I'd already seen. It had the same script, but with a "B-list" cast. With a resigned sigh, I half-heartedly rattled off my health history, past injuries, and ambitious goals, again emphasizing that weight loss was my top priority, no matter the cost.

For the first (but certainly not the last) time, Trainer #2 defied my expectations. Instead of just smiling and nodding, which would have been the easy way out, he actively engaged, patiently listening to everything I said. His insightful questions made me rethink my motivations and gently challenged some of my beliefs about health and fitness. Even with my stubborn resistance, he didn't give up, trying his best to connect with me and to understand where I was coming from, which was especially impressive considering I wasn't putting my best self forward.

Then, we reviewed the program I had been following with Trainer #1. With a refreshing level of honesty and confidence, Trainer #2 admitted it didn't quite align with his style and offered me a choice. I could stick with the old plan or try something new. It was a pivotal moment, a fork in the road.

Blinded by my not-yet-processed grief over losing Trainer #1, I didn't see this choice for the opportunity it was. All I knew was that hearing "Last set, best set!" from anyone else was enough to make me want to curl up into a ball and cry.

I had always been fiercely controlling when it came to my health and fitness. The "restrict and sacrifice" mentality gave me a false sense of control over whatever chaos was going on in my life, so I clung to that approach like I was holding on for dear life. But after losing Trainer #1, I was ready to give up. I had no fight left in me.

Uncharacteristically, I surrendered. I handed the reins over to Trainer #2, mumbling something about trusting his expertise and agreeing to do whatever he thought was best. That unwilling leap of faith turned out to be the right call. It was the catalyst that propelled me forward in my journey, even though it initially felt like a giant step back.

Trainer #2 wasted no time, putting me through a series of strength and form assessments that immediately gave me confidence in his abilities as a trainer. "Maybe this won't be so bad!" I thought, feeling cautiously optimistic.

That optimism was promptly extinguished when he handed me a workout plan that looked like it was designed to turn me into a She-Hulk. It may as well have been ripped straight from the pages of a bodybuilding magazine. And just like that, every one of my cynical prejudgments felt instantly, horribly validated.

My inner mean girl, seeing her opening, pounced on that "I told you so" moment like it was the last designer handbag on sale. "I knew he wouldn't get it," she couldn't resist pointing out, fluffing her imaginary boa.

I eyed the plan with a mix of disbelief and dread. "Is this guy delusional?" I thought. He clearly couldn't see the nearly forty-year-old woman standing before him, still trying to catch her breath from the epic stair climb to the gym.

My irrational dislike of Trainer #2, fueled by my grief over losing Trainer #1, colored our first few workouts. I basically gave him the conversational equivalent of a cold shoulder. It wasn't him, it was me. He was friendly and kind and even cracked some decent jokes that I stubbornly refused to find funny. The problem was that he wasn't Trainer #1, and that was enough for me to hold a grudge.

As the weeks rolled on, my initial resistance to Trainer #2 slowly started to melt away. It began with a grudging respect for his knowledge and expertise. The guy clearly knew his stuff. More than his impressive know-how, it was his endearing quirks that won me over.

He hated crooked barbells with a passion and would scour the gym for a perfectly straight one, like the slightest bend in the bar would throw off my entire workout. He also had an uncanny ability to trip over literally anything in the gym—weights, benches, even thin air—yet somehow recover with the agility and grace of a black-belt martial artist. And don't even get me started on his eagle eye for spotting the tiniest, rogue 2.5-pound plate from clear across the gym floor. It was like he had a superpower, a sixth sense for misplaced gym equipment.

I couldn't help but tease him mercilessly, and his good-natured responses and complete lack of ego about his quirks made him impossible not to like. We were an odd pair on paper, but built a genuine friendship that easily transcended our differences.

And to my astonishment, I *loved* my bodybuilding program. I was getting stronger by the week, and the feeling of adding more and more weight to the bar was surprisingly motivating. Trainer #2 typically had a very calm, relaxed vibe. But even he couldn't contain his excitement at my rapid progress. Whenever I added a few more pounds to the bar, you'd think I'd just won Olympic gold. His enthusiasm was contagious. It reminded me of the joy I felt as a kid playing sports, something I did simply for the love of moving my body without any pressure or expectations.

As it turns out, you can't judge a gym bro by his pump cover (that's the oversized shirt gym rats wear to hide how jacked they really are, for those of you not fluent in gym lingo!). I judged Trainer #2 harshly at first. However, the personal growth I experienced in those first few months of training with him was more than an unexpected surprise; it was a big step toward a much needed shift in my mindset. Instead of gritting my teeth until I reached my goals, I was starting to enjoy the process.

My goals were still miles away, but the thrill of tangible progress was undeniable. Trainer #2 and I were an unstoppable team. But as we all know, life loves a good plot twist, and the next one in my story was just around the corner. This challenge would test my resilience and force me to confront my deepest fears and doubts head-on.

Muscle Power, Mind Power Tip #13: My On-Again-Off-Again Relationship with the Elliptical

Let's talk about my old arch-nemesis, the elliptical. It's the humble piece of cardiovascular equipment I've been trashing for a good chunk of this book. To be clear, I understand that the elliptical isn't inherently evil. It's a perfectly respectable lower-impact machine that's especially pleasant if you have achy joints.

It became the villain in *my* story because of how I was using (or rather, abusing) it. It was my sole, sweat-drenched weapon in a misguided, calorie-obsessed war on fat. I was convinced that the more hours I spent "ellipting" (yes, I'm making that a verb!), the faster the fat would melt away. My tunnel vision was so absolute that I'd selectively tune out any information that challenged this belief, effectively blinding me to the more transformative potential of exercise beyond just the immediate burn.

My time with Trainer #1 delivered a much-needed, if initially unwelcome, education on how our bodies adapt and change. That's when I began to learn a fundamental, if inconvenient, truth. My beloved elliptical simply wasn't the fat-loss panacea I'd been conditioned to believe it was. Looking back, it's obvious that toward the end of our sessions together, my singular obsession with torching calories had become counterproductive and even started to backfire.

Why the betrayal, my dear elliptical?!

123

And yes, that's precisely why it earned its nemesis status!

It all comes down to adaptation. Let's use running as an example. When you go out for your first 5K run, your body might burn fuel like a gas-guzzling vintage muscle car. But do it consistently, and your body starts leveling up its efficiency. It gets better at shuttling oxygen around your body and producing energy. Essentially, it does the same work with less effort, which means fewer calories burned. Before you know it, you're breezing through your run with the energy efficiency of a hybrid car.

While this is fantastic for your endurance (and your carbon footprint), it's a big problem if your primary goal is fat loss. To keep seeing the scale move down, you need to constantly up the ante. You need to exercise longer or harder, you need to cut back on calories even more, or a combination of both. It feels like trying to outrun a treadmill that's secretly speeding up while someone's sneaking bites of food off your plate.

There's another major downside to excessive cardio, especially when you're under-fueling like I was. Your body, in its desperate search for energy, might start eyeing your precious muscle mass as an expendable resource.

Remember Trainer #1's borderline unhealthy obsession with protein?

It turns out that biology was firmly on his side. Without enough fuel, especially the protein crucial for maintaining, building, and repairing muscle, those long or intense cardio sessions signal your body to scavenge energy wherever it can. That's when muscle becomes a prime target. It's the metabolic equivalent of throwing your furniture into the fireplace to keep warm because you forgot to buy some firewood.

For the longest time, I just didn't *get* weight training. Why should I bother if my calorie tracker barely acknowledged its existence? If my elliptical marathons were a calorie-burning inferno, lifting weights was more like striking a match. It was a tiny, insignificant spark in comparison.

I thought the calorie burn was everything. But as it turns out, it's the *least* interesting, *least* impactful long-term benefit of exercise, and this is doubly true for weightlifting. The calorie burn during a strength training session is practically irrelevant, because the real payoff happens only *after* you put the dumbbells down.

While cardio primarily burns calories during the activity itself, strength training triggers a cascade of physiological processes that increase your metabolism long after you leave the gym. The more muscle you build and maintain, the more calories your body burns at rest, leading to a higher overall metabolic rate. The spark of weight training might not feel as powerful as the elliptical inferno, but it ignites a slow-burning, sustainable ember. It's not quite enough to grant you a free pass to gorge on pizza every night, but it is enough to make a difference in our modern world where we sit too much and calories are easy to come by.

Now, if you've spent any amount of time on the fitness side of social media, you've seen the short, attention-grabbing clips (and sometimes entire accounts) that love to pit cardio against weights, framing it as an either/or battle for fat loss supremacy.

This creates the illusion that you need to pick a side, which is a binary decision that leaves you feeling like you're missing out on *something*, regardless of which camp you choose. Sadly, that black-and-white thinking is more about generating clicks and controversy than providing nuanced guidance.

So, after all my wrestling with ellipticals and epiphanies about barbells, this is where I've landed. Both cardio and strength training are non-negotiables for me. I do cardio for my heart health and for sustained energy, and I lift weights for the bone density and muscle mass I need to live a long, healthy life (but also because I'm not mad at how great my shoulders look in a strapless dress!).

Finally grasping these concepts was huge for me. But the real surprise was what this process started to do for my head and heart. I didn't anticipate how my dedication to *"Muscle Power"* would become the very thing that rewired my *"Mind Power."*

Muscle Power Mind Power Tip #14:
The Heavy Lifting of Mindset Change

Thanks to Trainer #1's early efforts, I had a much more balanced routine, strategically weaving in foundational strength work and mixing up the cardio. It was a great starting point, and Trainer #2 ran with it. He took that foundation of strength training and made it a pillar of our work (much to the dismay of my inner mean girl, who was still convinced he was secretly trying to turn me into a She-Hulk). I knew that if I got the physical plan right, the results would follow.

But unexpectedly, Trainer #2 and I took it a step further by tackling one of my biggest limiting beliefs.

For most of my adult life, I'd treated my body like a never-ending, vaguely disappointing renovation project. Exercise was the joyless manual labor I had to endure to "fix" it. Every session was measured by calories torched, the number on the scale, or how I thought I looked in the mirror. It was a calculated, joy-sapping effort to correct my perceived flaws. Exercise had always been a form of self-inflicted punishment.

But as I progressed in my program with Trainer #2, something clicked. Weightlifting reminded me of playing sports for fun as a kid.

While skating like the wind from one end of the rink to the other during a ringette game, the thought of calorie burn never once entered my hyper-focused, nine-year-old mind. I did it

127

because I thrived on the exhilarating feeling that my powerful legs made me much faster than my teammates. I certainly wasn't analyzing my quad development mid-plié in dance class. I danced because it felt like expressing art through an enjoyable, physical challenge. Dancers are deceptively strong! And I sure as heck wasn't obsessing over how my stomach looked in the mirror during kickboxing drills. I did them because I knew they'd help me kick ass (literally and figuratively) in a sport I loved.

My adult brain had become so laser-focused on the metrics, and my head was buried so deep in my miserable "body renovation" project that I'd suffocated the intrinsic pleasure of movement. I'd forgotten that exercise could actually make me feel *good*. Trainer #2, with his patient guidance and focus on my abilities, helped me start digging my way back to that simple truth.

And when I allowed myself to shift my focus away from the grind and tune into how energizing, empowering, and just plain fun my new way of training felt, the stubborn fat loss I'd been so desperately chasing for years through punishment and restriction started to happen more naturally, almost as a pleasant, nearly effortless side effect of simply enjoying myself and feeling good in my own skin.

Ultimately, it wasn't my body that should have been the focus of my endless renovation projects. My thinking needed a *"Mind Power"* rebuild, starting from the bedrock up.

I used to roll my eyes when I'd hear one of those alarmingly cheerful fitness fanatic types chirp, "Just learn to love the process!" It always felt so disingenuous, and so dismissive of the teeth-gritting struggle. I didn't see my lack of love for the process as a problem, and I thought all I needed was the discipline to power through it.

I didn't realize that unhooking exercise from punishment would be one of my biggest *"Mind Power"* shifts, profoundly impacting my consistency and, ultimately, my results.

Joy. From *exercise*. Who knew? I certainly didn't see that one coming.

While finding joy was a breakthrough for me, your internal roadblock might be something else entirely. Maybe it's the belief that you don't have time, that you're "not an athletic person," or that you're destined to fail because you always have before (which was also classic Lisa!). Whatever your particular internal hurdles are, remember that the heaviest lifting is always in the mind.

When that internal resistance softens and your mind stops being an adversary, the effort you put into any goal (physical or otherwise) starts feeling like an act of self-care, with progress as its rewarding companion.

CHAPTER 8

Setbacks Happen

I t was early spring 2020, and life was good.

After finally finding my rhythm with Trainer #2, I was having a blast, loving the bodybuilder gym routine I'd initially resisted, and feeling stronger and more confident than I had in decades. Trainer #2 and I were smashing PRs (personal records, in gym speak!) left and right, and that made me feel unstoppable.

That was, until spring 2020, when the world seemed to hit pause with the first COVID-19 lockdown announcements.

Clearly, the universe felt that Trainer #1's injury wasn't the only lesson I needed to learn in adversity. So, it threw a pandemic-sized wrench into my perfectly sculpted plans, leaving me stranded in a bizarre alternate reality where toilet paper was a prized possession, hand sanitizer was liquid gold, and sweatpants were the new power suit.

I vividly remember that last workout with Trainer #2 before the gym doors officially slammed shut. We tried to stick to our usual lighthearted banter, but it was a flimsy attempt to cover up the mounting anxiety we were feeling. We finished the workout and exchanged a goodbye hug with a mix of optimism and uncertainty, offering up hopeful, if hesitant, comments about crushing leg day together again soon, utterly clueless that four long, gym-less months loomed before us.

As I headed to my car, I could feel the weight of the unknown pressing down on my chest. The second I slid behind the wheel, the tears came. More than losing the gym and the community I'd found there, I cried because I was terrified of losing all my hard-earned progress. I couldn't shake the question of what would happen to *this* new routine, *this* fragile momentum, and *this* progress that felt so significant yet still so new.

I had been steadily climbing upward on my fitness journey, fueled by a growing sense of self-efficacy and the thrill of pushing my limits. But resilience—the ability to adapt, bounce back from setbacks, and keep moving forward even when the world felt like it was imploding around me—was a muscle I was only just beginning to flex.

I was about to learn just how important that muscle would become.

It's funny how those old neural pathways, the old habits carved deep into our brains by years of repetition, never fully disappear. When uncertainty and stress close in, they can feel like a comforting escape. The gym hadn't even been closed a week before I was scrolling through my fast food app with practiced ease, shamelessly reuniting with my favorite delivery driver, the one I'd ghosted just a few short months earlier.

My inner mean girl smelled blood in the water and didn't pass up the opportunity to strike: "See? I knew you couldn't keep this up! You're weak, undisciplined, and destined to fail. Get out your stretchy pants... Because this isn't going to last!" A part of me believed her. I was afraid that I wasn't strong enough to maintain my progress without the structure and support of my gym routine and my coach. Bite by bite, I was proving her right by making that fear my reality.

I tried to keep my struggle under wraps by hiding my shame behind forced smiles and hollow reassurances. After all, binge eating thrives in secrecy. Thankfully, my brother, my ever-observant pain-in-the-ass roommate, had this annoyingly accurate radar for my emotional well-being. He knew I was faking it, even if I didn't have the guts to ask him for help.

Spring had arrived early in Canada that year. The unseasonably warm weather and sunny skies offered relief from the lockdown blues we were all feeling. One sunny April day, as I wallowed in self-pity on my favorite recliner, my brother burst into the room with an idea.

"Let's go for a bike ride!" he exclaimed, his enthusiasm matching the beautiful weather, but starkly contrasting my dreary disposition.

With nothing but reruns on TV and a world that seemed to be falling apart, I couldn't muster a decent excuse to refuse. "But... My allergies! The pollen count! My nonexistent knee injury!" I protested.

The truth is, I hated my bike. I'd bought it nearly a decade earlier with visions of carefree commutes, channeling my inner effortlessly fit and chic cyclist. But somewhere along the way, my bike had become a symbol of my struggle with food. Instead of enjoying windswept hair and the sun on my face, I'd forced myself to ride it as punishment for those moments when I'd lost control and binged, hoping to burn off every last shameful calorie. A tool meant for health and freedom had become tangled up in my unhealthy coping mechanisms.

Thankfully, my brother saw through my half-hearted excuses and practically dragged me off my comfy chair. The promise of post-ride pancakes was the only thing motivating me as I put on my cycling gear. With all the excitement of a trip to the dentist, I headed out for a ride. That day, I found myself dealing with two pains in my ass—my brother (in the most loving way possible) and my bicycle seat (which was decidedly less forgiving).

My initial reluctance to get back in the saddle was no match for the fresh air, the endorphins, and a healthy dose of sibling rivalry as my brother and I raced each other up hills. We were both morning people, but those sunrise rides turned us into a pair of obnoxiously chipper early birds. We explored every nook and cranny of our city, pedaling through sun-dappled parks, cruising down winding trails, and discovering other hidden gems we never knew existed.

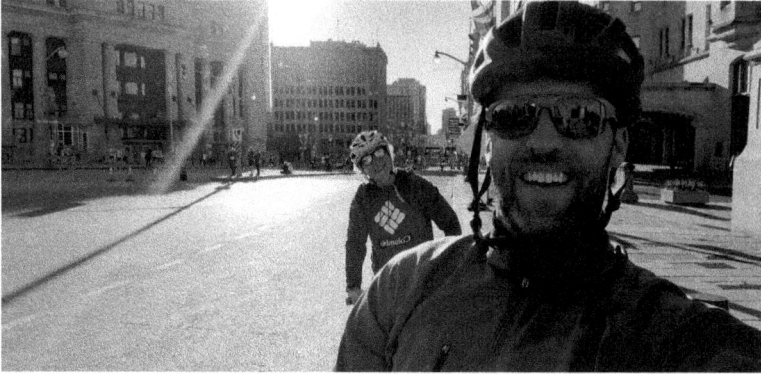

Lockdown partners in crime—2020 edition.

Time flew by as we chatted about anything and everything, a welcome escape from the constant barrage of bad news and chaos around us. By the time the lockdown restrictions finally eased later that summer, we'd logged enough kilometers to easily cover the distance between Vancouver and Halifax. But more importantly, those rides had chipped away at the darkness that had settled over me, reminding me of the simple joy of movement and connection.

I'm forever grateful that my brother and I were locked down together. It could have been an epic disaster, trying to navigate a global pandemic while cohabitating without driving each other crazy. But instead, we were partners in crime, cheerleaders for each other's struggles, and comedic relief in the face of a terrifying new reality. We had always been close, but those years under lockdown forged a bond that was literally strong enough to withstand an apocalypse. Our relationship was the silver lining in a very dark cloud, a reminder that there's always room for connection and laughter, even in the toughest times.

Meanwhile, Trainer #2 and I stayed connected with regular text messages. Inspired by my daily cycling adventures, I transformed my living room into a makeshift gym, with a random assortment of mismatched dumbbells, a few kettlebells, some neon resistance bands, and a yoga mat that had seen better days. Every other day, I'd sweat and curse through the modified workouts Trainer #2 thoughtfully adapted to my limited set-up.

As rumors of loosening lockdown restrictions filled the late-summer air, I could barely contain my excitement. Trainer #2 and I were texting up a storm, eagerly plotting our triumphant return to the gym and the familiar rhythm of our workouts. And because I'd clung to some semblance of my old routine during that first lockdown, refusing to fully surrender to my old "stagnant and flaccid" ways, we hit the ground running (or rather, lifting) the moment those gym doors cracked open again.

Over the next year, the pandemic became my unwitting resilience coach. Lockdowns came and went with alarming frequency, each one further testing my resolve. When the gyms reopened, each training session became a chance to dig deeper and challenge myself further. Every time the world threw another lockdown at us, I kept adapting, evolving, and finding new ways to keep moving forward. Time and again, my living room transformed into a gym, as I stubbornly refused to let uncertainty dictate my progress.

After each lockdown announcement and gym closure, I still cried in the parking lot. In fact, crying in my car might have been my 2020 version of self-care. But I also bounced back quicker every time. I learned that pain is unavoidable, but resilience allowed me to transform that pain into a source of power and growth.

Muscle Power, Mind Power Tip #15: Mind Over Mirror

Despite constant interruptions and less-than-ideal circumstances, my fitness journey had been quietly but steadily moving forward. Progress in the gym has a mind of its own, sneaking up on you when you least expect it. After a year of navigating the unpredictable landscape of pandemic life, my body finally caught up with my dedication, and the physical changes I'd been working toward were undeniable.

Because the pandemic had turned us all into stretchy-pants-wearing hermits, the comfy clothes that had become my wardrobe staples had cleverly concealed the changes that were happening underneath. It wasn't until one fateful day, as I pulled on a pair of pre-pandemic underwear that promptly slid off my hips and pooled around my ankles, that the reality of my transformation truly hit me.

With shock and delight, I raided the back of my closet, otherwise known as the graveyard of too-small "goal outfits", and triumphantly tossed one too-big item after another into a growing donation pile.

The woman in the mirror was a stranger. It felt surreal. I'd not only reclaimed my old wardrobe from the back of the closet but had also exceeded every physical goal I had ever set for myself. My reflection revealed a shape I barely knew. My collarbones had started to peek through. Just above my more narrow waist were the first hints of abdominal muscles. Even my legs, my biggest insecurity, were noticeably smaller.

I barely had time to reconcile what I was seeing before a familiar feeling crept in, crowding out the fragile feelings of satisfaction and pride. The strong, fit woman I had glimpsed only moments before vanished, replaced by a wave of dissatisfaction and self-criticism. Despite all my progress, my body still didn't align with an ideal I'd been chasing my entire life. It was like a flashback to my teenage years, trying on my graduation gown and feeling that pang of disappointment, that same sense that my body wasn't good enough. Once again, my past and present collided as an old insecurity I thought I'd buried resurfaced from the depths of my memory.

Suddenly, I was twelve years old again, sitting at a crowded restaurant with my soccer team after winning a big tournament. The smell of pizza and celebratory laughter filled the air, but all I could hear were the words of another mom. As I tucked into my meal, she leaned over to my mom to remark on my "sturdiness" and "healthy appetite." It was the 90s, and comments like that were sadly common, especially among women.

She wasn't cruel, so I know she didn't say it to be hurtful. She probably thought I couldn't hear what she was saying. But her words cut deep. My size had always made me feel different, a little out of place, like a giant outsider peering into a tiny world where I didn't belong.

The more I worked with Trainer #2, the stronger I got. In fact, I was getting *ridiculously* strong. I absolutely loved pushing my limits to see what my body could really do. But those words echoed in my head decades later because I could see that my training was also causing my body to change and, more frighteningly, *grow* in ways I hadn't anticipated.

Reflecting on it now, I realize why it was so hard to change my thinking. I had unwittingly bought into the belief that my worth was tied to my appearance, that smallness and thinness were the ultimate feminine values, and that strength and femininity were somehow mutually exclusive. It was a tough mindset to break, a deeply ingrained narrative that had shaped my self-perception for years.

I started to question whether I should keep lifting heavy weights. My inner mean girl, ever the opportunist, capitalized on my doubts. "If you keep lifting," she warned, "you're going to end up looking *big* and *manly*. You'll never have the *feminine* body you've always wanted."

Thankfully, I had Trainer #2 in my corner. He regularly reinforced my changing mindset with compliments on my strength and growing muscles. He'd say things like, "Your rear delts are popping!" or "Do you have any idea how *freakin' strong* you are?" He never used words like *thin*, *skinny*, or *small*, and it made all the difference. His focus on my ability starved the "thinness equals feminine worth" narrative my inner mean girl kept feeding me and opened the door to a whole new kind of self-worth—one that had nothing to do with the number on the scale or the label inside my jeans.

This feeling was far more valuable than trying to squeeze myself into some outdated cookie-cutter mold of what a woman "should" look like. I started feeling a sense of pride in the changes I saw, and a sense of ownership over my strength and power. Slowly, I stopped caring about labels like "manly" or "feminine."

I loved weightlifting and how it made me feel, and that was worth fighting for. So, with a defiant wink and a sly smile aimed squarely at my inner mean girl, I picked up a *ridiculously* heavy dumbbell and got to work.

Muscle Power, Mind Power Tip #16:
Showing Up Imperfectly

On my first day at the gym, as I climbed the winding staircase to meet Trainer #1, my inner mean girl was in rare form, ready to exploit every insecurity.

"You're not ready for this," she scoffed, preying on my lack of experience and knowledge. "You don't know what you're doing; everyone's going to laugh, and you'll fail like you always do," she added, dredging up memories of every diet I'd ever quit, and every exercise program I'd abandoned. "What will people think?" she taunted, amplifying my anxieties about being overweight in a gym setting. "They'll see you jiggling on the treadmill and laugh behind your back. And that outfit? *Seriously*? Is that what you're going with?"

And then, she unleashed her most potent weapon: "*Who do you think you are, even trying?*" This one stung the most, minimizing my goals and tearing away at the fragile confidence I'd mustered just to walk through those doors.

As cruel as my inner mean girl's words were, they held a grain of truth: I wasn't ready for a major life overhaul. Given the stress I was under, my emotional state, and my ongoing disordered relationship with food and exercise, the wrong clothes and shoes were the least of my problems.

I had the wrong mindset altogether.

My first steps were *far* from perfect. But by taking those steps, by simply showing up and trying, I had unknowingly challenged one of my deepest-rooted cognitive distortions, "all-or-nothing" thinking.

I was convinced that if I wasn't perfectly prepared, if I didn't meticulously plan every detail, if I couldn't control every factor, the only possible outcome was failure. It was an exhausting and unrealistic standard to hold myself to, but one I held tightly, believing that any deviation from the "perfect" path would lead to disaster. I thought this mindset would prevent failure, but as it turns out, it only made failure an absolute certainty.

Perfection is an illusion that keeps us frozen in place, convinced we need the perfect diet, outfit, playlist, and astrological alignment before we can even lace up our sneakers. But the courage to start, even when we feel like we don't belong, is far more valuable than waiting for the perfect moment—a moment that, let's face it, will likely never come. We'll always find something to hold us back if we're looking for an excuse. Ultimately, the messy, imperfect process of trying and failing and trying again pushes us to grow and learn.

This lesson was so good that I thought I'd learn it a second time, just for kicks.

Months later, when the pandemic hit, my inner mean girl saw her chance to stage a comeback, bursting back onto the scene with a vengeance.

"It's not the right time," she declared, capitalizing on the chaos and uncertainty. "It's too hard," she whined as the gym closures tore my carefully constructed routine apart. "Why bother? What's the point in trying when everything is falling apart?" she concluded, hammering her point home with a sense of finality.

And once again, she wasn't entirely wrong. The world was upside down, and my health and fitness goals felt trivial in comparison.

But then, my brother invited me to go for a bike ride. It was an unexpected detour, but I'm so glad I (begrudgingly) took it. During those crazy times, with masks and lockdowns limiting our interactions, connecting with my brother and clinging to a sense of normalcy felt far more important than any specific fitness goal. Cycling unexpectedly provided that and so much more. It may not have been "perfect," but it helped me maintain my momentum by preventing me from slipping back into old habits. More than that, it allowed me to make meaningful progress toward my goals despite the circumstances.

The open road offered a surprising clarity. It was as if the physical exertion cleared the mental fog, allowing me to see my inner mean girl in a new light. She wasn't the villain I thought she was, but a misguided protector, a scared child trying to shield me from feelings of pain and disappointment. Her voice echoed societal expectations and past traumas, attempting to keep me small but safe, even if it stifled my potential.

I'm still a work in progress, and my inner mean girl is a constant reminder of that. She'll always be a part of me. But instead of letting her negativity take me off course, I try to approach her with compassion, gently acknowledging her anxieties and reminding her that we're in this together. Her protests don't destabilize me like they did in the past. If anything, they've become a sign that I'm stepping outside my comfort zone, pushing my boundaries toward self-discovery and goals worth chasing. In that space of healthy fear where I'm constantly challenged and inspired to grow is exactly where I want to be.

CHAPTER 9

The UnDiet – My First Steps Toward Unlearning Diet Culture

By early 2021, a little over a year into my transformation, pandemic fatigue was really starting to set in. Gym openings and closures had become both an unsettling pattern and my new normal. But I was determined to keep the momentum going. Nothing would stop me.

Despite my imperfect routine, I'd lost 90 pounds. I was thrilled. Everything seemed to be falling into place. You'd think with all these positive changes in my life that I'd be bursting with energy and vitality, but the truth was far from it. I wasn't thriving. In fact, I was struggling.

I hit a sticking point where the scale stubbornly refused to budge for weeks, even though I was eating far less than I had at the outset of my journey, and nowhere near enough for someone of my activity level and build. To stick to my unsustainably low-calorie budget, I resorted to desperate measures reminiscent of my crash-dieting days—skipping meals, surviving on black coffee and diet soda, and white-knuckling my way through intense hunger pangs. My energy levels plummeted, which turned the workouts I loved into a grueling test of my willpower. My frustration was building, and worse, my body was sending me clear signals that something was seriously wrong.

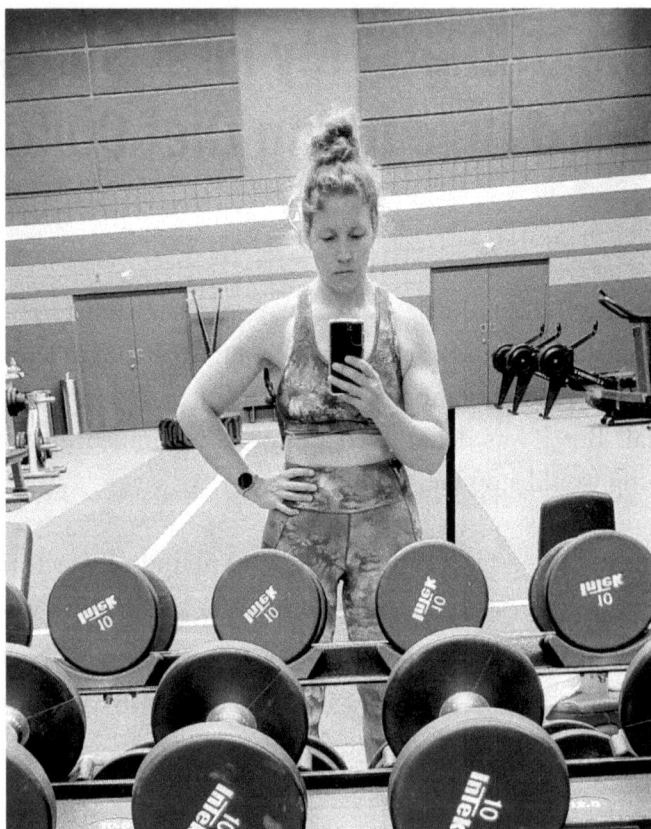

Chasing the "after" photo, but ignoring the internal warning signs.

The first signal was exhaustion. I'd always been a terrible sleeper, battling insomnia throughout my life. A little fatigue felt perfectly normal to me. But this was next-level, a bone-deep weariness that permeated every aspect of my daily life. My brain felt like mush, and I stumbled through my days in a fog. The fatigue also amplified my ravenous hunger, making it even harder to stick to my meager calorie budget.

As bad as the exhaustion was, the second signal was far more disturbing and devastating for someone as vain as I can be. My hair was falling out in handfuls, clogging the shower drain and leaving my once-thick ponytail feeling alarmingly thin. I tried to brush it off at first, but my rapidly thinning hairline wasn't buying it.

I frantically Googled my symptoms, only to discover the universal truth of the internet: If you have more than two symptoms, you definitely have cancer. Clearly, self-diagnosing on the internet wasn't the answer I was looking for.

Note: If you happen to find yourself relating to my story and are experiencing similar symptoms, I strongly encourage you to consult a medical professional (and I'm not talking about Dr. Google!) to rule out any serious underlying medical conditions.

That's exactly what I did, and the results were a bit of a mixed bag. While my lowered blood pressure and resting heart rate were encouraging, I was also essentially malnourished and deficient in key vitamins and minerals. My doctor promptly referred me to a professional. She possessed not only extensive qualifications in nutrition but also empathy that was rooted in lived experience. Crucially, she understood the dark side of dieting and disordered eating, which allowed her to recognize that this wasn't just about food but my whole relationship with eating and my body.

I felt seen and understood, finally in good hands. Together, we analyzed my test results, dissecting every detail. Then, she outlined a plan that was both comprehensive and surprisingly simple. As much as I wanted to trust her expertise, her primary recommendation filled me with dread.

She told me to eat freely without restriction until I felt *genuinely satisfied.*

Even though my eating habits had significantly improved, I was still actively recovering from BED. The word "satisfied" sent shivers down my spine. Satisfaction? That was a foreign concept to me, something I hadn't truly experienced in years of disordered eating. If I gave myself free rein to eat what I wanted, I knew what would happen. I'd eat to numb my emotions, to fill a void I couldn't even name, and to create a blissful fog of avoidance. It didn't make sense to me. The only possible outcomes? Regression. Relapse. A free-fall back into the abyss of binging. There's no way *this* was the solution I was after.

My voice trembling slightly, I voiced my concerns, revealing the depth of my fear and anxiety. To my surprise and relief, she was a compassionate ally, meeting my fears with understanding and validation, not judgment. We agreed it was time to step away from the rigid rules and restrictions that had become a part of my life. I would delete my calorie-tracking app, a constant source of anxiety and obsession. I would stop skipping meals, a practice that had left me feeling constantly hungry and vulnerable to binges. And most terrifying of all, I would reintroduce some of my "forbidden" foods back into my diet.

To be clear, she wasn't suggesting an all-you-can-eat Oreo buffet. She advocated for a whole-food approach, emphasizing nutrient-rich options while gradually reducing my reliance on processed foods. We explored the "plate method," a simple visual guide for creating balanced meals by dividing your plate into portions for protein, carbohydrates, and vegetables. It was a revelation, a way to make intuitive choices without obsessing over numbers. I'll talk more about these strategies in the next chapter, but they're simple, effective tools I still use today.

Beyond the "what" of eating, we also tackled the "why." Together, we explored the complex topic of hunger, emotions, and food cravings. She taught me to pause, listen to my body's signals, and distinguish between genuine hunger and emotional cravings. Remember that feeling of tension I would get in my chest when a craving hit? We learned to recognize the craving for what it was—a cry for comfort or a way to soothe stress or numb difficult emotions. It wasn't necessarily a demand for food. Acknowledging and observing my emotions without judgment often helped them fade away. And when cravings persisted, we explored healthier ways to approach them without resorting to restriction or punishment.

We talked about how food wasn't the enemy. Sometimes, eating a cookie or a slice of my mom's homemade casserole made with love was the most nourishing choice I could make. We discussed building a relationship with food based on curiosity, kindness, and self-compassion. She was the one who recommended I read the Josh Hillis book I mentioned earlier.

Our conversation extended beyond the plate to the realm of general health and fitness. She emphasized the importance of fueling my body adequately for my activity level, especially with protein, which was a message both Trainer #1 and Trainer #2 had struggled to get through.

This should have been a lightbulb moment, a wake-up call to prioritize my health over my weight that would set me on a path toward a healthier relationship with food and my body.

But I wasn't ready to give in just yet.

After all, I'd lost a whopping 90 pounds doing things my way, so surely I knew what I was doing. Despite the alarming test results, the advice of multiple medical professionals, and the distress signals my body was sending, I was clinging to the dangerous illusion that my harsh, unsustainable "restrict and sacrifice" approach was the only way. My fat loss success, ironically, had become an obstacle, blinding me to the possibility of a different, healthier approach. The idea of eating more food, of ingesting significantly more than the tiny calorie budget I'd been clinging to didn't just feel like a contradiction, it felt like a full-on betrayal of everything I'd worked so hard for.

Eating more had to mean gaining weight, didn't it?

It would take yet another intervention to finally break through my resistance and open my eyes to a new perspective. This time, the wake-up call wouldn't come from my brother, but from Trainer #2.

Muscle Power, Mind Power Tip #17:
The Mind Games of Cognitive Dissonance

I don't know about you, but when I was a kid, I believed my folks knew absolutely *everything*. They were the ultimate sources of truth and the keepers of all the answers.

My mom once told me that if you swallowed your bubble gum, it would stay lodged in your stomach for *seven years*. I lived in mortal terror of accidentally gulping down my Bazooka Joe.

One day in health class, my teacher explained the nuance of digestion. She casually mentioned that gum passes through like any other food, but perhaps at a more leisurely pace. With that explanation, the scientific reality of how my gut actually worked was in a head-on collision with my belief that my internal organs were accumulating years of indigestible rubber.

That feeling, that specific mental discomfort I experienced over a wayward piece of Bazooka Joe? That's the essence of cognitive dissonance. It's the destabilizing feeling as your brain scrambles to reconcile the conflict between what you believe to be true and the new, contradictory evidence. It can feel uncomfortable, even if the new information makes sense and your old beliefs are doing you a disservice. In this case, it presented as relief mixed with the dawning suspicion that maybe my mom didn't know *everything* about human biology.

It was a relatively harmless revelation.

151

But when the medical professional suggested I eat freely until I was "satisfied"? She may as well have told me the earth was flat, and that gravity was a government conspiracy. Her advice contradicted everything I believed about health, fitness, and, most importantly to me at the time, weight loss. This new information sent shockwaves through my brain, triggering a full-blown cognitive dissonance meltdown. My brain was screaming, "DANGER! This goes against everything we know! Abort mission!"

The funny thing about cognitive dissonance is that when faced with information that challenges our deeply held beliefs, our first instinct isn't polite consideration. We double down, becoming masters of justification. We'll twist facts, cherry-pick evidence, and find solace in echo chambers to support our beliefs. It all comes down to our brain's preference for the path of least resistance. It's infinitely easier to stick your fingers in your ears and hum loudly than to actually expend the mental energy required to do the work of changing your mind.

Overcoming cognitive dissonance isn't easy, but it starts with a simple choice. You have to be willing to get uncomfortable.

Challenge yourself to be curious. This means intentionally poking holes in your echo chamber. For example, if you're a die-hard low-carb fan, listen to a well-argued podcast episode defending the benefits of complex carbohydrates. You don't have to agree, but the first step is cracking the door open to a different perspective.

Especially when it comes to health and fitness, science and trends are constantly changing. What was considered absolute truth yesterday might be debunked tomorrow. My entire journey with strength training was a process of rewriting my beliefs about my body and its capabilities. Staying curious and open to new information is a crucial part of that process, allowing us to evolve and grow. It's important to challenge assumptions and remain open to new ideas and strategies.

So, the next time you run into information that makes your brain shout "DANGER!", take a breath before slamming the mental door shut. Recognize that feeling uncomfortable, defensive, or even irritated when your beliefs are challenged is totally normal. Instead of digging your heels in, try leaning into that discomfort with a little curiosity. Ask yourself honestly:

- Why does this bother me so much?
- What evidence supports my current belief?
- What evidence supports this new idea?
- Am I truly open to changing my mind if the evidence makes sense?

Give the other side a fair hearing in your own head. You might be surprised at what you discover.

Of course, this is me dispensing advice from the future. But back then, as we'll soon see, my "openness to contradictory evidence" skills were nowhere to be found.

Muscle Power, Mind Power Tip #18:
Building a Peaceful Relationship with Food

My ultimate nutrition goal has always been to eat more intuitively, like a *normal* person who wouldn't have a calorie counting app on their phone's home screen tallying up every bite that passes their lips, or a food scale permanently attached to their kitchen counter. But, as someone who had battled disordered eating for the better part of two decades, I had no idea what a *normal* portion size was, and my hunger and fullness cues were notoriously unreliable. Plus, with obesity rates on the rise, the definition of a *normal*-sized person or a *normal* quantity of food is constantly shifting, making *normal* a moving target that's not necessarily aligned with health.

So, I redefined my goal. I decided to eat in a way that aligned with my values and supported my fitness aspirations. I wanted to enjoy delicious food without guilt, have energy for the things I love, and prioritize my long-term health, all while building a sculpted, strong, and functional physique. If that sounds good to you, I'd like to share the strategies I use to this day to accomplish this.

1. Reduce ultra-processed foods

This is #1 on the list because it's so effective. Think about it. Factory-made treats are designed to be irresistible. Take the humble potato. Baked, it's a healthy, satisfying meal. But sliced thin, deep-fried, and coated in intense flavors, that same potato vanishes in seconds, leaving you with a lingering salty residue and an insatiable desire for more. That phenomenon actually has a name, "vanishing caloric density", a term for empty calories that don't satisfy and actually make you hungrier.

Ultra-processed foods overload your senses. Their intense flavors, enticing smells, and vibrant colors are a recipe for overeating. I love a good barbecue chip. The crunch, the salty-sweet-smoky explosion, and even the lingering dust on my fingertips is a calculated assault. The dreaded sugar-fat-salt combo triggers a dopamine rush in your brain, making it hard to resist another handful (or, in my case, the whole bag). It completely overrides your body's natural hunger and fullness cues.

There will always be a place in my diet for a peanut butter cup. But prioritizing whole, unprocessed foods keeps me full, energized, and satisfied, not to mention free from cravings or the processed food blues.

2. Abundance, not restriction

The word "diet" can make anyone feel deprived. Instead of thinking about what you can't eat, focus on adding goodness to your plate. Love peanut butter cups as much as I do? Here's how I make it part of my regular diet. Take a dollop of Greek yogurt, mix it with chocolate protein powder, and top it with a few mini peanut butter cups. It's a delicious, protein-packed treat that satisfies your cravings while supporting your goals. You can have a wonderfully satisfying, satiating, high-protein dessert for the same calories as your average-sized chocolate bar.

3. Make smart substitutions (or not!)

I love a good Starbucks Frappuccino, especially on a hot summer day. I'll treat myself to one from time to time, but they're calorie bombs. It's unrealistic for me to have one every day and still meet my health and fitness goals. Enter *Lisa's Favorite Protein Iced Faux-ppuccino* (recipe to follow)! It's my guilt-free, protein-packed version that satisfies my craving without derailing my progress. Finding fun and healthy substitutions for foods you love can be a nutritious and delicious experiment. In this case, Starbucks hasn't earned a cent from me since I came up with this recipe. It's an excellent substitution, and I don't miss the real thing at all.

But sometimes, substitutions just don't cut it. Making gluten-free, sugar-free, fat-free, dairy-free (and let's face it, probably taste-free) black bean brownies instead of your grandmother's mouth wateringly decadent recipe might not be the best idea. I'll eat the entire tray of "healthy" brownies and still want more. Sometimes, one bite of the real thing, savored slowly and mindfully, is much more satisfying than 100 bites of a brownie impersonator. Cravings can stem from a deeper desire for the sensory experience, the emotional connection, and the nostalgic memories associated with certain foods, like your mom's home cooking or a special holiday treat. Trying to replicate that with a healthified version can leave us feeling deprived, unsatisfied, and prone to overindulge.

Balance is key. Sometimes, a good substitute can hit the spot, but other times, exercising moderation and enjoying the real deal is precisely what you need. Find what works for you, your circumstances, and your body.

4. Eat slowly and mindfully

Eating slowly helps with digestion—which actually starts in your mouth! Chewing thoroughly breaks down food more effectively, making it easier for your body to absorb nutrients. In addition to that strategy, employing mindful eating techniques, like focusing on the flavors, textures, and aromas of your food, can also increase your enjoyment and satisfaction, making it easier to recognize when you're truly full and prevent overeating.

5. Eat until full, but not *too* full

Another skill to master is stopping at eighty percent full. This *hara hachi bu* concept from Okinawa, Japan, encourages intuitive eating and respecting your body's needs. I wish I could take my own good advice, but I struggle with this one because I like the feeling of fullness at the end of a meal.

That's why the next tip is a lifesaver for me.

6. The plate method made easy

The plate method was one of the most effective and surprisingly simple strategies I learned to create balanced and nutritious meals. Imagine your plate divided into three sections:

- *Protein*: One-quarter of your plate should consist of lean protein sources like chicken, fish, beef, tofu, eggs, cottage cheese, or Greek yogurt.

- *Carbohydrates*: Another quarter is dedicated to carbohydrates, such as whole grains like quinoa, brown rice, whole-wheat bread, starchy vegetables like potatoes, sweet potatoes, or corn, or beans, peas and lentils (collectively known as *pulses*, which are a great source of fiber-rich carbs, and as an added bonus, provide a decent amount of protein!). You can also include fruits in this section.

- *Non-Starchy Vegetables*: The remaining half of your plate should be filled with colorful, non-starchy vegetables like broccoli, cauliflower, spinach, kale, carrots, peppers, and zucchini.

This visual guide ensures you get a good mix of macronutrients (protein, carbohydrates, and fats) and essential vitamins, minerals, and fiber. Fattier cuts of meat, sauces, and other additions to your plate can often account for the fat you need, but this method also allows for some additional healthy fats, like a drizzle of olive oil, avocado slices, or a sprinkle of nuts.

I love the plate method because it's flexible and adaptable to any meal or cuisine. Everyone's having pizza? I grab a slice, load up my plate with a big salad, and add some extra chicken. This works at restaurants, too. My boyfriend and I often share an entree, and I'll order a side of steamed vegetables or a salad to round out my meal.

To ensure I feel full and satisfied, I always keep some veggies in the fridge, ready to be tossed in the air fryer and added to my plate. Cruciferous vegetables (broccoli, cauliflower, Brussels sprouts—you name it, I love it!) work exceptionally well. When

I'm doing my weekly meal prep, I blanch and then cool them, so all I need to do is crisp them up for a few minutes.

This ties in nicely with my final tip.

7. Set yourself up for success.

I'm definitely more successful at making progress toward my goals when I have a plan. Every Sunday, I dedicate about four hours to preparing a week's worth of breakfast, lunch, snacks, and a few family dinners. My go-to dishes include hearty casseroles like cabbage rolls and stuffed peppers, soups like my version of my mom's chicken and dumplings (recipe to follow), and vibrant stir-fries. I also use my slow cooker and pressure cooker to batch-cook proteins like tender pulled beef, pork, or chicken, that become the base for tacos, quesadillas, and burritos.

This four-hour investment is a trade-off I'll gladly accept for the stress-free and time-rich week it affords me. It also helps me reduce food waste, as knowing there's a delicious meal waiting in a neatly packed container makes me less likely to cave and order takeout when I'm tired or stressed. Plus, it saves me the embarrassment of having to explain to my favorite delivery driver why I ghosted him...again!

An unexpected bonus of meal prepping is that my boyfriend's adult kids have embraced it. They love my healthier versions of freezer burritos, vegetable mac and cheese, and chicken chow mein, and will reliably pick my "fakeout" options over takeout. In fact, my stepson's long-time girlfriend, a fixture in our blended family, asked me if I would create a family cookbook, and my heart nearly burst with pride.

Remember, these are just suggestions, tools in your nutritional toolbox. Find what works for you and your lifestyle. Pick and choose the tips that resonate with you, and ditch the rest! The goal is to create a system that supports your health and fitness goals while fitting seamlessly into your daily routine, a system that's sustainable, enjoyable, and uniquely yours.

Muscle Power, Mind Power Recipe #1: Lisa's Favorite Protein Iced Faux-ppuccino

Ingredients

- 80-100g of ice
- 180g of unsweetened vanilla cashew milk
- 1 scoop of protein powder
- 2 tsp instant coffee powder (to taste)
- 1 medjool date

Instructions

- Combine the ingredients in the order as listed above, and blend.
- Add optional toppings like whipped cream, chocolate chips, or chocolate or caramel syrup.

Notes

- Find your sweet spot with ice, and how it blends with your protein powder.
- I like cashew milk because it's very low in calories, and I pick the unsweetened vanilla version to add to (not overpower) the other ingredients that contribute to its amazing flavor. 180g gives me the perfect consistency, but use as much as you need to produce a creamy result.

- It's so important to love your protein powder for this recipe. I use whey protein powder (not isolate) because I prefer the texture. It makes my shake light, creamy, and fluffy. I've used vanilla, chocolate, salted caramel, and even maple donut flavored whey protein powder with outstanding results.

- I use espresso instant coffee for that extra coffee taste, and sub in the decaffeinated version if I'm having it later in the day so I don't sacrifice my sleep quality.

- Do yourself a favor, and use medjool dates in this recipe. Any date is fine, but the texture and taste of medjool dates is worth the effort. They taste like smooth, silky brown sugar. If you don't have a blender that will appropriately pulverize your date, soak it in a little hot water for a few minutes first.

This shake is my go-to pre-workout snack. I love it for the hit of caffeine from the coffee, the high-quality protein from the whey powder, and the quick carbohydrates from the date.

Muscle Power, Mind Power Recipe #2: Donna's Famous Chicken and "Dumplings"

My mom makes the dumplings, chicken stock, and bechamel sauce from scratch. Her soup tastes like a big, warm hug from grandma. Mine tastes more like a firm handshake—still thoughtful, but decidedly less personal. It gets the job done, tastes great, and takes a fraction of the time to prepare. The gnocchi is a surprisingly effective substitute for dumplings!

Ingredients

- 1 cup diced celery (100g)
- 1 cup diced carrot (125g)
- 1 cup diced onion (150g)
- 3 tsp minced garlic (15g)
- 1 tsp salt
- 1 tsp onion powder
- 1 tsp rosemary
- 1 tsp thyme
- ½ tsp black pepper
- 1 bay leaf
- 1 big rotisserie chicken, diced, skin and bones removed
- 2 cups chicken broth
- 2 cans of soup (284 mL each)
- 1 package potato gnocchi (454 g)

- 1 cup frozen peas (225 g)

- Parsley (it's just for looks, so fresh is best, but dried is also pretty!)

Instructions

- Put everything except the chicken, gnocchi, peas and parsley in the slow cooker. Cook on low for 4-6 hours, until the vegetables have softened.

- Add in the chicken, gnocchi and peas, and cook for another 30 minutes or so, until the gnocchi is ready.

- Remove the bay leaf.

- Ladle into bowls, and top with parsley.

- Notes:

- I use the lazy minced garlic in a jar. But if you're feeling ambitious, fresh garlic tastes so much better.

- Instead of a rotisserie chicken, you can use around 1 Kg (2.2 lbs) of chicken breast or thigh, cook it in the crockpot and shred with two forks.

- For the soup, I suggest cream of chicken, celery or mushroom. You can use low fat soup if you'd like, or even make your own bechamel sauce with flour, butter and milk.

CHAPTER 10

Trainer #2 (Part 2) – You Are An Athlete

On some level, I knew I needed to eat more to regain my health and rebuild my relationship with food. But I was desperately clinging to the familiar "restrict and sacrifice" mentality, the one that had led to my impressive weight loss. Feeding myself felt like venturing into a minefield of temptation and inevitable weight gain.

"You aren't actually going to listen to this terrible advice, are you?" my inner mean girl lamented, dramatically clutching her non-existent pearls. "This is the quickest way back to where you started, 90 pounds heavier. *Put. The. Fork. Down!*"

My brain could understand the logic, but my heart and gut couldn't let go of what they believed to be true. This was a textbook case of cognitive dissonance, and it would take two key insights to finally shift my perspective on nutrition for good.

Insight #1

As the gyms reopened in the spring of 2021 after yet another pandemic closure, I was excited to get back to my familiar training routine. Eager to share everything I had learned about nutrition and my eating habits with Trainer #2, I launched into a passionate monologue before I even did my first rep.

Trainer #2 listened patiently, nodding as I rattled off everything I'd learned about whole foods, protein, and proper fueling. He let me have my big "aha!" moment, graciously validating the very insights he'd been trying to drill into my head for months. I could practically see the thought bubble above his head: "She's *finally* starting to get it!"

But unfortunately, I didn't quit while I was ahead.

I carried on, outlining my plan to incorporate this new approach while maintaining a strict caloric deficit to lose more weight. I spoke with a frantic desperation, the kind that says, "I know what I'm saying is crazy, but please, for the love of all that is holy, tell me it'll work." I needed Trainer #2's support and validation to silence my internal turmoil. Blinded by that desperation, I couldn't read the room and completely missed the not-so-subtle shift in his expression, from agreement to concern.

Although he had earned my trust and the right to call me out on my self-sabotaging BS, he delivered his reality check in his signature kind and caring way. He placed a comforting hand on my shoulder, stopping me mid-sentence and grounding me in the moment.

With a reassuring smile and the kind of calm conviction that should be bottled and sold, he said, "You know, it's okay to *not diet.*"

insert screeching record noise here

The idea of not dieting felt absurd, and even a little dangerous. I hadn't not dieted since the late 90s. What would not dieting even look like for someone like me? My inner mean girl was ready to pounce. "I knew it," she scolded. "Back to square one, just like I predicted!" Her voice was patronizing, confident I was already headed down the well-trodden path to my nearly 300-pound former self.

But Trainer #2's words had already slipped past my inner mean girl's insecurities, and started dismantling the whole operation from the inside out. With those words, Trainer #2 had given me something I desperately needed.

Permission.

I'm not talking about permission to stop dieting. It was more profound than that. He gave me permission to stop battling myself. Permission to let go of the rigid rules and restrictions I had clung to for so long. Permission to listen to my body, to trust my intuition, and to nourish myself without guilt or shame. Permission to choose a path that aligned with my health, happiness, and values.

Trainer #2's words, filled with agency, freedom, and the promise of a different way of living, gave me the courage to open myself up to a new perspective, and try something new. My inner mean girl was rendered speechless.

And just like that, her decades-long winning streak was over. I had finally chalked up a win.

I wish I could say that it was smooth sailing from there, but there are two hard truths about transformation that can't be ignored.

First, change rarely happens overnight. Unlearning the decades of ingrained beliefs about food and my body, and dismantling the negative self-talk that had ruled my life, was a slow, often painful process. Week by week, I increased my calories by adding more whole foods to my diet, allowing myself to eat until I was full and satisfied. I leaned heavily on meal prepping to keep me on track, ensuring I always had healthy options on hand, especially when life got busy.

Second, change rarely goes smoothly. Even though I knew better, my inner narrative still defaulted to the familiar, and my opportunistic inner mean girl was always ready to act at the first sign of weakness. "Ugh, another week of meal prep? Where's the fun in that?" she'd whine. "Are you sure this is sustainable? You're going to get bored and fall off the wagon again."

Stepping outside of my comfort zone was terrifying. The unfamiliarity of this new approach made me question whether I could succeed. My worst nightmare was that I would fail and end up proving my inner mean girl right. My progress meant everything to me. I couldn't bear the thought of losing it all and ending up back where I started, or worse, heavier and more discouraged than ever. The stakes felt impossibly high.

Thankfully, Trainer #2, my wise coach and supportive friend, stepped in a second time. His insightful guidance offered another much-needed perspective shift. This missing piece would put me squarely on the path to cementing these changes for life.

Insight #2

Trainer #2 did his usual check-in at the start of one of our training sessions, asking about my sleep, energy levels, and how I was fueling my body. Parroting the words of my inner mean girl, I started ranting about how sick I was of eating the same boring foods every day.

"I feel like I'm eating like a dog," I grumbled.

Without missing a beat, he shot back with a grin, "No, not like a dog. Like an *athlete*."

"*Athlete?*" I scoffed. "With all due respect, I'm pretty sure they don't hand out Olympic medals for fat loss!"

After we shared a good laugh, Trainer #2 took the time to explain his perspective. He talked about how athletes eat with intention, understanding that every snack and every meal has the potential to help them perform at their best. What he was saying made sense, and if adopting an "athlete mindset" could somehow make broccoli taste a little less like freshly mowed lawn, then I was willing to try it.

My resentment around my food choices vanished. I had finally started to see how prioritizing nutrient-dense options aligned with my goals and supported my active lifestyle. I even got creative with meal prep, finding combinations that made my pre-packaged meals genuinely enjoyable. In no time, the workouts I loved started to feel good again as I regained my strength and confidence in the gym. And all it took was eating food I enjoyed while fueling my body for performance like an athlete would.

The rest of 2021 was a time of learning and unlearning, discovering what worked best for me, my body, and my lifestyle. I learned that progress requires flexibility, a willingness to adapt my strategies to fit my life. But most importantly, I realized that fat loss was just one part of the wellness picture. As my focus shifted from shrinking my body to building a strong and healthy one, my motivation deepened, and those old, destructive patterns weakened until they lost their hold on me.

On New Year's Eve, I took a moment for my usual end-of-year self-reflection. For so long, I had been playing the same losing game, following the old rules of restriction, deprivation, and self-sabotage. But Trainer #2 had handed me a whole new playbook, one based on self-compassion, a more intuitive approach to eating, and fueling my body for performance. I wasn't battling myself, I was building a better me, inside and out. And with that, I had finally achieved a level of health and fitness success that had eluded me for over two decades.

It was a new year with a new focus, and it all started with a single step up those gym stairs. "Stagnant and Flaccid Lisa" had faded into the background, and "Lifting Lisa," stronger and more confident than ever, was the one calling the shots.

I smiled with pride as I reviewed my resolutions for 2022. For the first time in my adult life, my resolutions reflected a deeper desire for personal growth, strength, and living a life that felt authentic and fulfilling.

Weight loss? It didn't even make the list.

Muscle Power, Mind Power Tip #19:
Breaking Up with the "Old You"

Eighteen months after our split, my ex-husband and I decided to grab lunch. There were things we needed to talk about and sort out. We hadn't seen each other since the day I dramatically tossed my belongings out the window of the condo we once shared, like a scene from a rom-com gone wrong. Our incompatibility aside, our marriage had been happy, and we were on friendly terms. Despite feeling a little anxious, I was genuinely looking forward to seeing him.

It's funny how you can live your own transformation every single day without truly seeing it. The accumulation of subtle changes can be practically invisible to the one who experiences them. But then you're confronted with someone from your past, and suddenly it feels like you're in a time warp, simultaneously living in the present while being pulled back into who you were.

My ex-husband was exactly the same as the last time I saw him. He was still the witty, intelligent, kind-hearted guy I'd married, but seeing him felt like looking at a perfectly preserved artifact. He was a poignant link to my "before," and piece of my past that hadn't changed, and that stillness highlighted the change in me. The woman who had dramatically tossed her belongings out the window and sped off to "The Roach Ritz" ("La Cucaracha Inn?" "The Pest-ige Suites?" I could do this all day!) was a stranger to us both. She was a different person, a character in a story I had outgrown.

I still hold a special place in my heart for "Stagnant and Flaccid Lisa," who rocked a well-worn Metallica t-shirt, subsisted on takeout, and considered the fast-food delivery guy a close friend. She got me through some dark days, and I owe so much to her stubborn resilience.

But to step into this new chapter, I had to do the unthinkable and break up with her. I had to let "Stagnant and Flaccid Lisa" go.

Breaking up with yourself, even when you know it's for the best, is a bit like cleaning a closet. It always gets messier first. Picture a full-on internal soap opera. There were floods of tears (mostly in my car, my signature move for processing difficult life events), dramatic accusations of betrayal, and my inner mean girl throwing the kind of epic, metaphorical door-slamming tantrum that would make an angsty teenager proud.

But this was a necessary process that allowed "Lifting Lisa" to emerge. She was stronger, self-assured, confident, and more aligned with my true self. The person I had become, with healthier habits, a brighter outlook, boundless self-belief (and let's not forget, killer biceps!), felt infinitely more authentic than the old me ever did.

It was through this messy process of breaking up with myself that I stumbled on a trick for creating lasting change.

Instead of dreaming about the person I want to be, I get in her head. I think through her priorities and the habits and the actions she takes to fuel them. By understanding her values and motivations, I can start making those same choices for myself immediately. We've already talked about how fake-it-till-you-make-it doesn't really work, but this is more like practicing your way into a new reality. The distinction is about authenticity. Faking is a performance; practicing is a process of becoming.

For example, when I decided to write this book, I didn't just tell myself "I am an author," and hope for the best. I actively stepped into the role of "Literary Lisa." She had a demanding job, a family, a relationship, and responsibilities she couldn't ignore. But she carved out the time, even if it was only stolen moments between other commitments. She set boundaries around her writing time, fiercely protecting it as a priority because she knew that consistency is key. She did that, day after day, week after week, for over two years until she was done.

The result is that "Literary Lisa" triumphantly nailed her lifelong dream of writing a book. Beyond that personal victory, she also found that sharing her story opened the door to meaningful connections with others, which was a way of honoring and living out her values. It's a true win-win.

So, who is the "new you"? Are you "Veggie Vivian"? "Zumba Zoe"? "Nature Nat"? "Boundary Beth"? "Self-Care Sarah"? Or maybe you're "Powerlifting Patricia" or "Marathon-Running Maria"?

Picture her. Imagine her life in vivid detail. Feel her energy, her confidence, and her passion. Then ask yourself the following questions:

- *How can you bridge the gap between who you are now and who you want to be?*

- *What changes need to happen in your life to align with her values and priorities?*

- *What habits and behaviors does she embody that you need to cultivate?*

Make those behaviors, habits, and actions yours. Don't just dream about her. Choose to become her *now*.

Muscle Power, Mind Power Tip #20:
The Biggest Loser Curse

Remember that infamous reality TV show, *The Biggest Loser*?

Airing in 2004, *The Biggest Loser* captivated millions with its promise of dramatic, rapid weight loss. Led by celebrity trainers who pushed contestants through diabolical workouts, the show offered the ultimate fantasy for anyone struggling with obesity. Check out of your life, lose a ton of weight, and win a pile of cash. Back then, the idea of fully immersing myself in shrinking my body at that ranch was pure, dream-come-true material.

The show's aftermath revealed a far less inspiring reality. Countless contestant stories highlighted an uphill battle to maintain that dramatic progress. Many regained most, if not all, of the weight they'd worked so punishingly hard to lose. But why did these individuals who seemed to have every advantage and resource at their fingertips struggle so deeply to keep the weight off?

While the sweaty, tear-filled journey of losing weight gets all the glory and airtime, losing weight is just Phase One. The consistent work of weight maintenance is the criminally overlooked Phase Two.

The data paints a stark picture that supports the experience of many *Biggest Loser* contestants. The overwhelming majority of people who lose significant weight gain most, if not all, of it back within a few years. It's not a failure of willpower, but a testament to the physiological realities of adaptation and the psychological toll of extreme restriction.

This sobering reality hit me like a ton of bricks, because I saw myself in those contestants' stories. Just like them, I was running on fumes, eating far too little to sustain my energy, my sanity, or my results. My approach was a textbook recipe for rebound weight gain. I knew with gut-level certainty that if I didn't change now, their "after" story would become mine.

I couldn't allow that to happen. I was determined to break the *Biggest Loser* curse. This meant finally listening to Trainer #2 and embracing the deeply uncomfortable, counter-intuitive idea of not dieting by actively fueling for strength and, dare I say it, maybe even *growth*.

Ugh. Easier said than done after a lifetime obsessed with shrinking.

To make that shift stick, my goals had to change. This new direction inspired my 2022 New Year's resolutions, which refreshingly abandoned the tyranny of the scale in favor of a healthy relationship with food and my body. With a new focus, the next chapter of my journey revolved around three simple yet powerful guiding principles: *Eat well, get strong, and enjoy life.*

CHAPTER 11

Trainer #2 (Part 3) – Eat well, and get strong!

It was early 2022, and with the new year came a renewed sense of purpose. I was excited to sit down with Trainer #2 to discuss my goals. Transitioning to weight maintenance felt like a new world was opening up, with the chance to sculpt my body by strategically building muscle.

I wanted to start with my legs. My loose skin was a visible reminder of the weight I'd lost and a source of insecurity. I understood that after two decades of being overweight, my forty-year-old skin would never snap back to its pre-weight-gain tightness, at least not without a scalpel and a long recovery. I had realistic expectations. We had nothing to lose by trying to improve the appearance of my legs through muscle gain.

Next on my list was my butt. Genetically, I have big legs and a flat butt (thanks, dad!), and I was determined to prove that a bubble butt could, in fact, exist in my family lineage.

And finally, I wanted to build my shoulders. I always felt like they sloped into my arms, with no shape or definition, and I was ready to change that.

The game plan was twofold: Balance out my pear shape by building broader, rounder shoulders for a more hourglass silhouette, and fill the loose skin on my legs with lean, strong muscle. With our new goals set and a new program in hand, we got to work, training hard and smashing PRs like we always did.

To kick off my weight maintenance and muscle growth phase, I took a long, hard look at my dietary habits. I knew tracking my food intensely, as I had done in the past, would be a slippery slope back to restrictive eating and the obsessive mindset I was working so hard to overcome. I decided to continue with the more intuitive approach to eating I had been using. But since building muscle was a priority, I also needed to ensure I was eating enough protein.

So, I settled on a compromise. I tracked my protein intake while trusting my body's signals for everything else. It was the perfect middle ground, allowing me to ensure I was getting enough protein for muscle growth while still honoring my hunger and fullness cues. It meshed well with the "plate method" of eating, which I absolutely loved. I consistently hit my protein targets while still enjoying delicious meals with family and friends, leaving the table feeling satisfied, not deprived.

Since I didn't want to restrict any foods, I adopted a simple rule to keep my notorious sweet tooth from feeling deprived. I would allow myself to indulge in homemade treats made with love, but pass on the pre-packaged stuff (unless it's movie popcorn or a peanut butter cup!). It was a sustainable and enjoyable way to balance my cravings with my values, and ultimately, my goals.

You'd think that eating more would have been a piece of cake, a celebration of food freedom. But that wasn't the full story. There were also some challenging downsides. Let's start there.

I knew that as my body adjusted to the increased food intake, I was bound to gain some weight. Even though I felt energized and was crushing it in the gym, I couldn't ignore the subtle signs that my body was changing. Once comfortably loose, my jeans now hugged my thighs and hips in a way that screamed, "Maybe lay off the extra protein, okay!?" The increasingly snug fit of my jeans became a source of anxiety, a reminder of the weight I'd lost and the fear I had of regaining it.

The scale was becoming a problem too. Every morning, I'd eye it in the corner of my bathroom, my anxiety mounting with every ounce I gained.

Of course, my inner mean girl was having a field day at my expense. "Your jeans are screaming for mercy! Can you even breathe?" she said. When her voice taunted me, I wrestled with the urge to revert to my old ways and white-knuckle my way through another "restrict and sacrifice" diet. "A few days of rabbit food, and the scale will be back to normal in no time!" my inner mean girl prodded, tempting me with the promise of a quick fix.

I reminded myself (repeatedly) that I needed to trust the process. I was playing the long game, and wanted to fuel my body, not starve it. So, I banished the scale to the closet for the sake of my well-being. Then, I reluctantly bought some new jeans with a little wiggle room. It was a small concession, a symbolic surrender to the fact that my body would keep changing. But it was also a giant leap toward self-acceptance and embracing a new definition of what it meant to be healthy and strong.

Comfort and confidence became my new mantras as I navigated this unfamiliar territory, trusting that my body would find its happy place with a little patience and a lot of self-love.

With the "downs" out of the way, let's move on to the glorious "ups"!

Social eating became infinitely easier. Gone were the days of agonizing over restaurant menus, obsessively counting calories, or feeling deprived while everyone else indulged. I embraced mindful eating, savoring the foods I wanted in quantities that satisfied me, not stuffed me. Friends would marvel at my "whatever I want" approach to eating, including dessert, if it appealed to me. Their eyes would widen with envy and disbelief as I enjoyed my food with genuine pleasure and zero guilt. "I could never do that," they'd say, shaking their heads and nibbling on their sad salads (hold the dressing).

Sometimes, I'd try to explain that this lifestyle was attainable with a balanced approach that included regular exercise and focused on whole, unprocessed foods. But that was a tough pill to swallow, especially for people who had the same ideas around food and dieting as I used to have. I'd often just smile and accept their compliments on my "fast metabolism." It was a secret wink to myself, knowing it was the hard work of consistency and discipline, fueling my body appropriately, and a lot of sweat equity that got me there.

I rediscovered the joy of cooking as I breathed new life into old family recipes by adding protein and veggies to our comfort food classics. I used the plate method to create balanced, satisfying meals, ditching the measuring cups and calorie calculators. Mealtimes with my loved ones became a celebration of good food and good company, leaving everyone feeling nourished and content.

Finally, after many months of trial and error, I reached a comfortable equilibrium. I felt good about my eating habits, my workouts were a blast because I had energy to spare, and I was starting to love the way I felt in my own skin. It seemed like the perfect time to check in with my old friend, the bathroom scale. To my surprise, I was back at the weight I had started from.

Curiosity piqued, I decided to track my calories for a few weeks to see what was happening. To my astonishment, I was averaging 2,800 to 3,000 calories a day to maintain my weight, which was nearly double the calories I was eating to lose weight. Online calculators for someone like me (185 pounds, 5'8", female, mid-40s, moderately active) suggest a maintenance level of around 2,260 calories. The adaptability of the human body, especially when you finally stop treating it like the enemy, is truly amazing.

But the most exciting part wasn't the number on the scale. It was the subtle but still undeniable transformation my body had undergone. My waist had shrunk from 32 inches to 29 inches, confirming that even though my weight remained constant, I was losing fat. My skinny jeans still didn't fit, but for the best reasons imaginable—my waist was too small, and my butt was too big. A "gym girl" booty requires a special kind of stretchy jeans, which was an expense I was all too happy to incur.

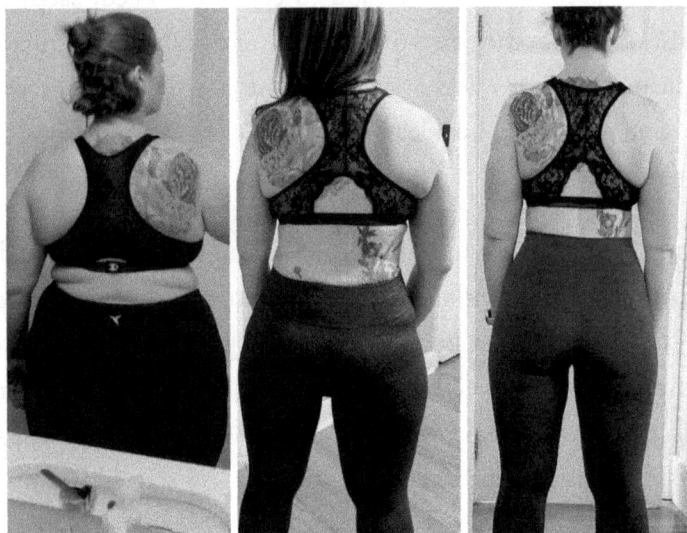

The evolution of my backside.

I saw similar changes in the rest of my body, too. My shoulders, which used to slope downward and disappear into my arms, had broadened and rounded, permanently retiring my blazers to the back of the closet. I didn't mind, because I finally had the hourglass shape I'd always dreamed of. Even my legs looked firmer and stronger, the underlying muscle giving them a more solid shape.

Eating more, maintaining my weight, and reshaping my body simultaneously? How does that even work?

The answer is body recomposition.

Body recomposition implies losing fat and gaining muscle at the same time. Fitness gurus will tell you to pick a side—fat loss (which requires an energy deficit) or muscle gain (which requires an energy surplus). They'll argue that body recomposition is "suboptimal", and that splitting your focus between the competing goals of fat loss and muscle gain is a surefire way to stall your progress.

And you know what? They're not wrong.

Focusing on a single goal is the most efficient path to progress. But as someone recovering from an eating disorder, the recommended "optimal" approach wasn't a great fit. Cycling through fat loss and muscle gain phases felt like it would mimic the binge and restrict cycle that had been so damaging. My approach allowed me to build a healthier relationship with food while gaining some muscle, and with it, plenty of strength and confidence in the gym. It certainly wasn't "optimal"—seeing even the tiniest, incremental changes took more than two years of dedicated effort—but it was the right call for me given the reality of my life at the time.

So, what did my training look like during this muscle-building phase?

You might expect a radical overhaul, but surprisingly, not so much. As it turns out, the kind of weight training that builds muscle is pretty much the same training you do while working toward a fat loss goal.

Instead of drastically changing my workouts, we focused on periodization—a fancy term for cycling training variables like volume, intensity, and exercise type—and adjusting my workouts to match the ebb and flow of my life. In the summer, when my mornings started with bike rides with my brother, we focused on improving my cardiovascular capacity and dialed back the weight training to two to three full-body gym sessions a week to maintain the muscle I'd already built.

During the holidays, when I knew I'd be eating more and indulging in treats like my mom's drool-worthy peanut butter, butterscotch, and marshmallow squares (seriously, you haven't lived until you've tried them), we'd crank up the intensity in the gym to direct those delicious calories toward building muscle and strength. It was a targeted but flexible approach that allowed me to enjoy life without sacrificing my fitness goals.

Before we go any further, I need to pause here to tackle the big, muscular elephant in the room. "But Lisa," I hear you ask, "with all that hardcore weight training and all those calories, didn't you get *bulky?*"

Nope. *Not even close.*

That's the short answer. Now for the long answer.

Muscle Power, Mind Power Tip #21: Your Ticket to a Toned and Empowered Physique (Not Bulkville)

From the moment I started writing this book, I knew sharing photos was non-negotiable. My story is raw and personal, and I wanted you to see the journey, not just read about it, so you can connect with my experience.

Easy decision, right?

I wish! Cue the internal meltdown.

My inner mean girl, who has an uncanny radar for vulnerability and a special talent for sabotage, strutted onto the scene: "Pictures? Of *you*? Who's going to relate to *that*? You're *too big* and *too muscular!*" For a second, she almost convinced me to scrap the whole idea because my version of "after" wouldn't resonate, and my transformation wasn't aspirational enough.

My "after" photos might not fit the standard 90-pound weight loss mold. I'm good with that because it reflects the deliberate evolution that took place. My initial, punishing goal of "get as lean as possible through intense food restriction and incinerating calories" gave way to the much more intentional focus of "repairing my relationship with food and my body by eating for performance and building muscle." What mattered most was achieving that healthier, stronger way of being. I was prepared to be happy with whatever shape my body decided to take as a result.

187

That shift alone completely rewrites the visual story.

Today, after a lot of *"Mind Power"* work, I wear my muscles with pride. My physique isn't an accident, it's by design. It's the result of years of dedicated strength training, consciously crafted because I fell in love with lifting and the incredible feeling of being *ridiculously* strong. And let's be clear, the amount of effort I pour into lifting these days far exceeds what's needed for general health and strength, and is lightyears beyond what I would recommend to someone just starting out.

So, let's see what years of dedicated strength training looks like in real life, outside the gym. Take a look at my "after" photos—say, the one of me on the beach, not-so-casually posing in my bikini:

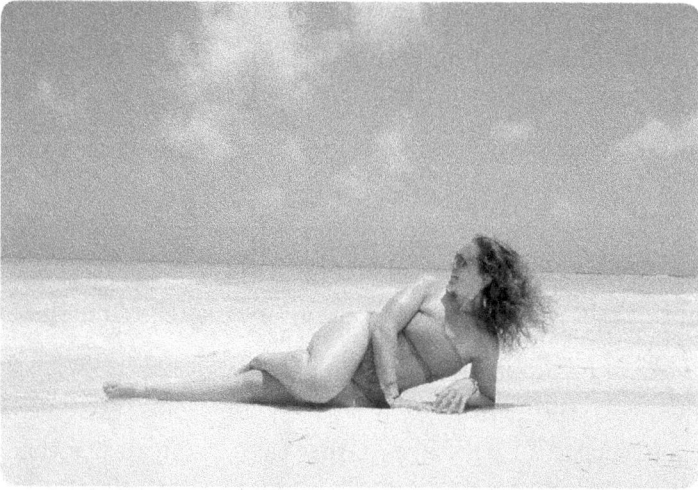

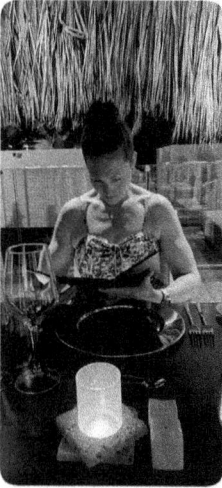

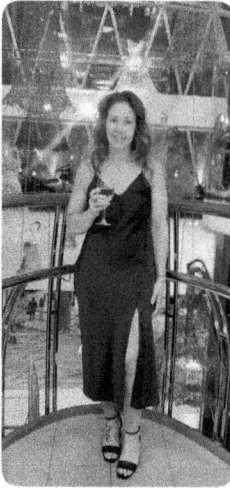

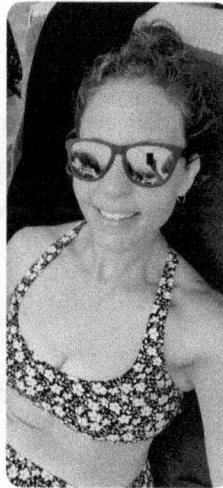

Built by consistency, fueled by strength.
Finally feeling at home in my skin!

If you didn't know my backstory, would your first thought be, "Is that a bodybuilder on vacation?" Or would you just see a woman who looks healthy and confident, enjoying a beautiful day on the beach?

Suppose you saw me wearing regular clothes, picking up a few essentials at the supermarket. Would you think, "Whoa! Did a professional strongwoman just ask me where the eggs are?" Or would you just see a woman trying to remember to pick up the toilet paper, like the rest of us?

By looking at me, you might guess I know my way around a set of dumbbells. But am I "bulky"? Not quite. And the idea that picking up weights two, maybe three times a week will accidentally turn the average woman into some kind of she-Schwarzenegger? I wish it were that easy. The reality is that no matter how hard I train or how much chicken breast I eat, I'll never wake up with a set of biceps that could crack walnuts.

I recognize the fear of getting bulky in so many women. I see it when they approach me in the gym, curiously peppering me with questions about my routine. Inevitably, the whispered concern comes next: "But I don't want to get as muscular as you." I always smile, because the unspoken implication is that my physique, the one I've poured years of sweat, effort, and strategic eating into, could somehow be achieved by accidentally stumbling into a vat of protein powder while doing a barbell squat or two.

I can't judge them for having that perception. It wasn't that long ago that I was worried about the same thing. So, I offer a reassuring smile and the same words I wish I could have said to my past self: "You don't need to worry about that. I've been trying to get bulky for years. Trust me, it's not a mistake you make—it's a full-time job. You're safe, I promise."

Strength training isn't a one-way ticket to "Bulkville." It's your express pass to a toned, capable, and empowered physique. It's the most effective tool for sculpting your body in a way that aligns with *your* goals. You'll get stronger, feel more powerful, and see a few muscles pop that you didn't know existed.

Building muscle allowed me to strategically shape the areas I wanted to emphasize, like my glutes and shoulders, while fat loss revealed definition elsewhere, like my waist and even my face. In those places that grew stronger and fuller, like my quads and hamstrings, the new muscle dramatically improved the appearance of my loose skin and cellulite, creating a firmer, more sculpted look. I didn't suddenly have the flawless derriere of a 20-year-old fitness model, but the changes were encouraging enough that I happily reinvested the money I'd half-jokingly stashed away in my "nip/tuck" savings fund right back into more personal training sessions with my coach.

Score one for the dumbbells and zero for my limiting beliefs!

If you're on a quest for a body that looks good and functions even better, you won't get it through hours of "ellipting." You'll get it with a weight that makes you work for it, whether that's a barbell, a dumbbell, a stretchy resistance band, or even your own body weight. The key is that it needs to challenge you, and over time, you need to challenge it back by bumping things up. While those adorable one-pound pink neoprene-covered dumbbells are a fine place to start, they eventually need to retire to Barbie's Dream House so you can pick up something even just a little heavier to signal to your muscles that it's time to grow.

Don't be afraid to push your limits and build that muscle. After all, the toned look everyone talks about is the visual proof of the strong muscle you built *underneath* the fat you lost. You gotta build it to show it!

CHAPTER 12

The Muscle of Gratitude

We all have those days. The ones where you feel stuck in a rut, convinced you're not making any progress. The days when a surprise ambush from your inner mean girl triggers a bad body image day, making even your favorite outfit feel about as flattering as wearing a brown paper bag.

I've had more than my fair share of those, especially wrestling with body image throughout my transformation. I've learned that on those "throw in the towel" days, it's time to hit "replay" on my personal highlight reel.

Every now and again, a feel-good moment would materialize when I least expected it but needed it most. These weren't big, earth-shattering events but small, significant interactions where someone saw something in me that I was struggling to see in myself. Without being asked, these strangers who became acquaintances and sometimes friends would offer a kind word or a moment of connection. They recognized my strength, my spirit, or just my stubborn willingness to show up and do the work, often reflecting back a better version of me than I felt at the time.

The stories that follow are moments frozen in time that still fill me with warmth and remind me I'm moving in the right direction. I hope that by sharing them, you'll not only find pieces of your own experience reflected here, but also be inspired to recognize and cherish your own "highlight reel" moments. Inspiration and motivation are contagious, and passing it on is what this is all about.

1. The InBody Scan Surprise

One day, as I walked into the gym, I noticed a booth set up so members could get InBody scans—fancy machines that measure weight, muscle mass, body fat, and more. It had been a while since my last one, so I decided to give it a shot despite being a little nervous about what the results would reveal.

A trainer I hadn't met before was working at the booth. I approached, and he invited me to step up and start the assessment. As the results slowly materialized with the whir of the printer, my heart sank when I saw my weight coming into view.

It was higher than I expected.

But before I could catastrophize and turn this moment into a major freak-out, the trainer grabbed the printout. He quickly scanned the results, and his jaw dropped. With an incredulous look on his face and his finger pointed squarely at the measurement of my muscle mass, he blurted out:

"You're as strong as *fuck!*"

My disappointment melted away as we burst into laughter.

2. The Jacked Guy at the Gym

By late 2022, the gym felt like home. I had been a fixture there for long enough that I started to become familiar with many of the gym regulars. There was this one lean, muscular guy I would always see, no matter when I showed up at the gym. If he told me he worked out twice a day, seven days a week, I would have believed him. His physique reflected that level of dedication. You could easily use his chiseled body to teach a muscular anatomy class.

In my head, I always referred to him as "Ridiculously Jacked Guy."

One day, I was pushing myself hard on the glute drive (a butt-sculpting machine). I worked my way up in weight and still felt I could do more. As I was standing there, contemplating increasing the weight again, I noticed "Ridiculously Jacked Guy" trying to get my attention.

I removed my headphones, and he asked, "Can I work in?" I smiled and agreed. Pointing at the weight loaded on the machine, he said, "You're a beast. I don't even know if I can get this!"

I was brimming with pride.

He did his set and watched in awe as I added more weight to the machine and did mine. We laughed, bonding over our mutual love of lifting.

We're gym friends now.

3. I Need to Put My Shirt Back on...

Not every day was a perfect day in the gym. Sometimes, my workouts sucked. The dumbbells felt heavier than usual on this day, and my lifts weren't going well. Frustrated, I considered bailing on my workout halfway through. Mid-spiral, I turned around in surprise as a fellow gym-goer tapped me on the shoulder.

"I've gotta hand it to you... You're absolutely jacked!" he exclaimed. "I had to put my shirt back on before coming over here to talk to you!"

His kind words were a much-needed boost, especially during a terrible workout. I thanked him for taking the time to walk over and say that to me, if only to make me feel good about myself.

We're also gym friends now.

4. Glute Sisterhood

I was working on a heavy set on the leg press machine when I noticed this girl doing hip thrusts with an inhuman amount of weight on the bar. I couldn't help but watch as she locked out four perfect reps.

When she finished, I walked over to tell her that she was my gym hero. She smiled and replied, "Coming from you, over there killing it on the leg press, that means a lot!"

It turns out she was also watching me.

You guessed it, gym besties for life.

5. Strength Inspiration

I was doing a set of Romanian Deadlifts, one of my favorite lifts. Headphones on and music pumping, I was locked in. I knocked out eight perfect reps, racked the weight, removed my headphones, and settled in for a well-earned rest.

The woman training beside me looked over and said: "You're *so* strong. It's inspiring!"

I want nothing more than for other women to experience the strength and confidence that weightlifting offers. That comment made my year. I smile and wave at her whenever I see her at the gym, knowing that every workout brings her one step closer to experiencing that feeling for herself.

6. The Compliment That Almost Wasn't

My legs were on fire as I finished a particularly punishing set of walking lunges. As I dropped the weights and steadied myself with a few deep breaths, I saw a personal trainer I knew walking over to say hi. But instead of his usual greeting, something completely unexpected came out of his mouth.

"You're looking beefy!" he said.

Caught off guard by his comment, a flash of my old self flickered, suddenly terrified of looking "too bulky."

"You know," I found myself saying, "if you said that to any other woman, she'd probably punch you in the face!"

He chuckled, commenting over his shoulder as he walked away, "Guess I'm lucky you're not any other woman then!"

While "beefy" might not be the adjective every woman dreams of, in the context of years of hard work and a deliberate goal to build strength and visible muscle, it was a genuine, unvarnished compliment. He saw *power*, he saw *dedication*, and he saw *results*. My mindset had shifted so much that instead of recoiling, I could actually hear and appreciate the admiration in his voice.

I finished the rest of my workout with a smile on my face.

7. Training the Trainers

We were midway through a solid upper-body session. Trainer #2 had me doing face pulls, really focusing on that upper back squeeze. As I pulled the rope toward my face, another trainer I know pretty well ambled past, did a double-take and pointed at my back, letting out an impressed, low whistle.

Before I had the chance to process that, Trainer #2 grinned at him and said, "I know, right? She'll be training us soon!"

I'm pretty sure I snort-laughed and almost dropped the rope. Beneath the embarrassment and the laughter, I was beaming. To have not one but two experienced trainers openly admiring the muscle I'd worked so hard to build?

That kind of validation was pure gold.

8. We're not worthy!

This last story is my favorite.

Trainer #2 was coaching me through some deadlifts. That day, the weight felt light, so we kept increasing the load on the barbell. It was going so well that we decided to push for a PR.

It was a huge goal, and I was feeling the pressure.

Hands shaking with adrenaline, I walked up to the bar for my big moment. Another trainer and his client paused what they were doing to watch my attempt. With Trainer #2 taking a video and the others cheering me on, I set up and pulled with everything I had. I locked out a perfect rep and let the bar fall triumphantly to the ground in an obnoxiously loud clatter.

Trainer #2 was so excited that he mindlessly tossed his phone aside and ran over to give me a big congratulatory hug. After we savored the moment, we retrieved his phone from the floor where it landed, and queued the video to watch it back.

What did we see in the background?

At the top of my lift, you could see the other trainer's client in the background, doing the "we're not worthy" bow from *"Wayne's World"*! If you're around my age or if you love iconic 90s movies, you know exactly what I'm talking about.

It's not every day I get to out-lift a human anatomy chart, earn a "strong as *fuck*" badge of honor, or have someone bow down to my deadlift prowess, *"Wayne's World"* style. So when it does happen, I lock them away in a special place in my heart reserved for these happy moments.

So keep lifting, keep laughing, and who knows? Maybe one day, you'll be the inspiration for a "we're not worthy" from a fellow gym-goer. And when that happens, take the time to bask in it— because you've *earned* it.

Muscle Power, Mind Power Tip #22:
Enjoy Life!

O n that happy note, I want to discuss the last of the three key areas that transformed during my maintenance phase.

Learning to enjoy life.

The sneakiest cognitive distortion, especially when it comes to any significant life change, is "I'll be happy when..." This was a favorite for my inner mean girl, who wouldn't hesitate to say things like, "Happy? You want to be *happy*? Sure, you can be *happy*... after you've lost at least another 20 pounds."

The "I'll be happy when..." way of thinking puts your life on hold, making your joy conditional on some elusive future goal. It's a never-ending waiting game, a blindfold that hides the beauty and joy that exist right now.

This is different from the "finding joy in the process" idea that we chatted about earlier. Finding joy in the daily grind of meal prep or a grueling workout might never happen for many of us. Sometimes the process is just that—something you commit to with determination rather than delight. But when you give yourself permission to soak up the good stuff already present in your life, like a belly laugh with a friend or the taste of your morning coffee, regardless of what the scale says or how "on track" you feel, you're building a more joyful existence for yourself, starting today.

With that in mind, let me tell you about a moment that changed my approach to enjoying the present.

Pretty early in my maintenance phase, my boyfriend and I planned a romantic getaway to the Dominican Republic. Even though the scale didn't reflect my "ideal" weight, I consciously left my insecurities at home with my winter coat. "Vacation Lisa" was going to be a confident queen. So what did I do instead? I stuffed my suitcase with nothing but bikinis. I even packed a thong.

You heard me, a *thong*.

In my tiny swimsuits, I spent the week strutting my stuff hand in hand with my boyfriend on the beach. I felt lighter than air, not once giving a second thought to the cellulite on my ass. The only thing on my mind was whether to enjoy my afternoon mojito next to the pool or on the beach.

I even did something I'd avoided for decades. My skills at avoiding having my picture taken had reached ninja status, so when a local photographer approached my boyfriend and me for a beachside photoshoot while we were on a catamaran excursion, my default programming screamed, "Run!" It was a reaction honed by years of perfecting my disappearing act.

Feeling the joy of that moment, I chose to be *in* the picture and capture the happiness instead of letting insecurity steal the memory. Choosing presence over my usual pattern of avoidance was a liberating experience. Because I made that choice, I have hundreds of gorgeous photos with the man I love, capturing our happiness in that stunning, exotic location.

They're treasures I'll cherish forever.

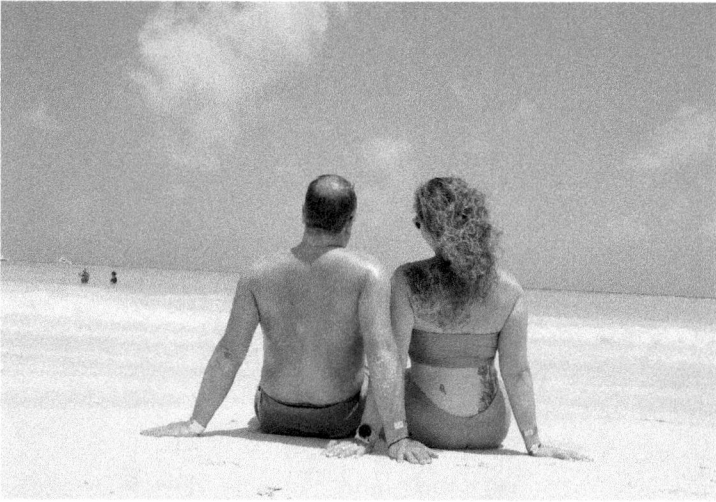

*Sunshine, sailing, Serge, and the moment I finally
said YES to the photo. Pure Dominican bliss.*

Living a full life means embracing the present while working toward the future. So, if you take anything from this part of my story, let it be this.

Embrace your journey, with all its ups and downs. Celebrate the small victories, the moments of growth, and the courage and strength it takes to show up for yourself. Give yourself permission to be happy now, not "when," because happiness isn't something you have to earn. It's woven into the fabric of your life, waiting to be savored in every moment and should never be held hostage by your goals.

And above all, you are magnificent, capable, and worthy, *just as you are.*

CHAPTER 13

Trainer #3 (Part I) – Embracing Change… Again!

It was late 2023, and Trainer #2 and I were at the end of a workout that had already pushed my limits. As I braced myself for the grand finale, the universally dreaded Assault Bike (yes, it's as torturous as its name implies!), Trainer #2 dropped some unexpected news that hit harder than any high-intensity interval ever could.

With a shaky voice, he revealed that he was stepping away from personal training. He had been offered a new opportunity outside the fitness industry, a career path that promised the work-life balance that working twelve hours a day, six days a week in a gym could never offer. At 29 years old, he was ready to step into his life, for a relationship, and maybe a family. Given the nature of the health and fitness industry, it's a difficult choice many trainers face, but wish they never had to.

I understood, of course, and I was also genuinely happy for him. Our friendship had grown to the point where I loved him like family, so I only wanted the best for him. As I offered my heartfelt congratulations and encouragement, I couldn't stop my voice from shaking a little, too. Even though the rational part of me knew I'd be okay, it still took everything I had not to burst into tears on the gym floor.

I held it together for the last few minutes of our session (thank you, Assault Bike, for making the pain in my legs a welcome distraction from the pain in my heart!), packed up my gym bag and headed to my car.

Slumped behind the driver's seat, I did what any self-respecting car crier would do, and let the floodgates open. Even though the repeated episodes of crying in my car might indicate otherwise, I had come a long way since the tantrum I threw after Trainer #1's injury and the rollercoaster of gym closures during the pandemic.

That's because this time, the tears weren't fueled by a fear of failure or a lack of self-belief. They were for my friend, the bond we'd formed, and the bittersweet realization that it was time for us to move on to the next chapter of our lives.

And what a chapter it had been.

Trainer #2 had been there for me through every hardship, every lesson learned, and every victory. He was a constant source of knowledge, support, and encouragement. The words "thank you" felt so small and insignificant compared to the enormity of his impact on my life, but it was all I had to give.

But it was time to decide what was next for me.

I knew I was capable. My progress—the early mornings, the meal prep, the relentless mindset work—was all my own, the result of grit and consistency. The old narrative that I needed someone else to facilitate my success felt demonstrably false, which inevitably led to a big, looming question.

Now what? Did I actually *need* to keep investing in a personal trainer?

In purely practical terms, the answer was no. After four years, I could hold my own in the gym. Plus, the things I loved most about it, like camaraderie, accountability, and support, I could get in other ways. Whether it was an online program with supportive communities, group fitness classes, even just training with a friend, there were plenty of ways for me to succeed with a much lower price tag.

But *need* and *want* often live on two different planets.

I deeply valued the structure and accountability a good trainer provided. In contrast to my usual control-freak tendencies elsewhere in life, it was a refreshing change of pace to show up and follow their lead. Letting someone else map out the plan, knowing they had my best interests and goals at heart, took a significant mental load off my shoulders. It freed me up to relax, embrace the challenge, and enjoy the process of pushing my limits.

So, despite having suffered the sting of not one, but two cases of "gym heartbreak" at the hands of brilliant coaches who became important fixtures in my life, I decided to open myself up and seek out that partnership one more time. It was time to find the next person who would believe in me, push me, and support me in becoming the strongest version of myself.

Trainer #2, who always had wise words to share, was the first person I turned to. He immediately suggested working with Trainer #3 as if it were the most obvious thing in the world.

Me? I wasn't so sure.

I knew Trainer #3 mostly by reputation, but I'd also caught glimpses of him in action at the gym. When I showed up a little early for my training sessions to warm up, he was often there, putting two of his Paralympic athletes through their paces. They were inspiring women, underdogs turned champions, thanks (I'm sure at least in part) to Trainer #3's guidance and expertise. I'd also heard that he was coaching a group of personal trainers from our gym in the finer points of Olympic lifting (which is the highly technical act of tossing insanely heavy barbells over your head and catching them like it's no big deal). From where I was standing, he had a formidable intensity and a dedication to performance that made me question if he even slept—or blinked.

Intimidated? Let's just say I was suddenly very interested in the location of the nearest fire exit.

I wasn't an athlete chasing podiums. I was a "lifestyle client" who still wrestled with my old emotional baggage. How could I, with my history of gym meltdowns and goofy jokes between sets, possibly measure up or be taken seriously by someone who trained *actual champions*? Sure, I could throw a heavy weight or two around, but my inner monologue during a workout was less "Eye of the Tiger" and more "Please don't let me drop this on my foot" or "Is it snack time yet?" It felt like a total mismatch, the fitness equivalent of bringing a spork to a knife fight.

For the second time in our relationship, I questioned Trainer #2's sanity.

Experience taught me that his seemingly crazy suggestions often led to unexpected breakthroughs. After all those years of training together, he knew me well—when to push, when to pull back, and most importantly, when I was ready for a new challenge, even if I was too stubborn to admit it. After all, it was his crazy idea to train like a bodybuilder and ditch dieting that led me to the healthiest, happiest version of myself.

Hesitantly, I decided to take his advice and reach out to Trainer #3. But instead of feeling excited about my new chapter, I felt resistance, like my gym sneakers were suddenly glued to the floor. Despite all the personal growth, there were still some unresolved emotions lingering under the surface, threatening to hold me back.

Muscle Power, Mind Power Tip #23: Battling the Imposter Within

It's clear now that this had been slowly building, waiting for the right trigger to unleash its full force. But to understand why this particular meltdown hit me so hard, it helps to know how significantly my life had changed in the years leading up to it.

The physical changes from all my hard work in the gym were remarkable, but they were dwarfed by the confidence and discipline I built. This internal transformation permeated every facet of my life, allowing me to build a successful career, improve my relationships with friends and family, and feel like my true self in a healthy and happy romantic partnership. But because my personal growth had been so unexpected and so fast, the life I was building felt precious and fragile, like a sand castle that could be swept away at any moment.

Losing Trainer #2 and having to start over with Trainer #3 shouldn't have been a big deal, but it was in this context. Just like before, it wasn't a major life event that triggered the meltdown; it was a tiny gym problem. But this particular tiny problem was the opening my inner mean girl had been waiting for, giving her all the fuel she needed to ignite an emotional wildfire.

Let me paint a clearer picture of how it all unfolded.

I was comfortable with Trainer #2, and maybe even complacent. He had seen me at my worst and had witnessed the struggles, tears, and triumphs. He knew my history, my insecurities, and my deepest fears. And somehow, he still believed in me.

But Trainer #3? He didn't know me. He was a blank slate. His fresh eyes felt less like an opportunity to grow and more like a spotlight, ready to expose every flaw I'd tried so hard to hide in the "new me." It threw me back to my first day at the gym, slowly trudging up the winding gym staircase—unemployed, broke, separated, and living in "The Roachmont Suites" (last one, I promise!) with my brother. That's when the fear surfaced, sharp and immediate.

What if Trainer #3 saw right through me?

That one question started a cascade of insecurity, and it wasn't long before the "what ifs" began to pile up:

- What if all my hard-earned gains in the gym evaporated under his critical gaze, proving "Lifting Lisa" was nothing more than an inspiring story I couldn't live up to?

- What if "Lifting Lisa" and the new life she represented— the career success, the happy relationships, all of it—was just a fragile lie, ready to shatter and reveal no real change had ever truly stuck?

- If he saw through the act, what if everyone else did, too? My boss, my friends, my family, my partner… how long would it be until they all realized I had never stopped being "Stagnant and Flaccid Lisa"?

As the tiny, hairline crack in my armor opened wider and wider, my inner mean girl backed up her metaphorical dump truck to unload a lifetime of dirt onto my emotional grave. Her words weren't new. They were the culmination of a lifetime of negative self-talk.

"Are you still trying to pull this off? The "Lifting Lisa" charade? Do you think you belong in this gym, with that career success, in that happy relationship? *Please.* It's all just an act, isn't it? You're terrified someone will see the real, insecure you hiding under all those layers. Trainer #3 won't be fooled by your fancy gym clothes or your fake, carefully practiced confidence. He will spot the fraud the minute you inevitably start fumbling, and everything will come crashing down."

It was imposter syndrome, pure and simple.

Imposter syndrome is the persistent, nagging fear of being "found out," of people realizing you aren't as bright, capable, or deserving as they thought. It thrives on insecurity and erodes self-confidence, making you question every achievement. Hard-earned successes become "flukes," and any well-deserved recognition or praise is obviously "luck" or people being nice because they haven't seen the *real* you yet. It exploits your fear of failure, your need for validation, and your beliefs about your worthiness.

To me, imposter syndrome felt like an unstable Jenga tower of all the cognitive distortions I struggled with. Every fear, every doubt, every "not good enough" was another block added to the teetering stack, threatening to collapse the whole structure at any moment.

It was a battle I hadn't anticipated hitting this hard, but maybe I should have. It's all too common, especially among successful people, and sadly, we rarely talk about it openly. Imposter syndrome can be particularly tough on women, because we're often conditioned from a young age to downplay our accomplishments, criticize ourselves, and prioritize others' needs. This creates the perfect environment for imposter syndrome to take hold and grow.

To anyone looking in from the outside, I was "Lifting Lisa," the confident, successful woman who had transformed her body and life. Shouldn't that accomplishment have been objective proof, protecting me from these feelings?

You'd certainly think so.

But the negative beliefs I held about myself—the ones that told me I wasn't good enough, strong enough, or deserving of my success—didn't magically melt away along with the body fat I'd lost. In fact, the dramatic, rapid transformation that happened in my body and life somehow amplified the feeling that I hadn't truly earned it. A stubborn part of me remained stuck in the past, leaving the door wide open for "Stagnant and Flaccid Lisa" to waltz back into my life.

Imposter syndrome thrives on emotional reasoning, a cognitive distortion that convinces us our feelings are facts. This dangerous mental shortcut tells you that because you feel a certain way, it must be true, regardless of any evidence to the contrary. We mistake our subjective feelings for objective facts, allowing the fiction of imposter syndrome to feel convincingly and devastatingly real.

To move forward, I had to change that narrative. Instead of believing the lies my inner mean girl was spinning, I had to replace them with empowering truths grounded in evidence. I needed to internalize that "Stagnant and Flaccid Lisa" was no longer my reality but a ghost conjured by years of negative self-talk. It took guts to confront my fears and insecurities and acknowledge how I was holding myself back. But leaning into that vulnerability is precisely where we open the door to genuine self-love and acceptance.

For me, that came through a surprising experience with none other than Trainer #3.

CHAPTER 14

Trainer #3 (Part 2) – When Awkwardness Leads to Awesomeness

M y imposter syndrome, I quickly learned, was about so much more than my gym anxieties. This pattern of self-doubt impacted my confidence across the board, from second-guessing my successes at work to affecting how I showed up in my personal life. Unraveling this emotional mess wasn't going to happen overnight, but grasping the "why" behind it gave me just enough courage to take the next step.

In late 2023, I contacted Trainer #3. His prompt reply reflected his professionalism, and we booked a trial session to see if it was the right fit for both of us. He told me to prepare for a leg day.

I *love* leg day.

It felt like a promising start.

Once again, I found myself at the foot of the now-infamous grand staircase at my gym. A chorus of worries filled my head with every step toward the gym floor. The gym had become my happy place, and the thought that the wrong coaching dynamic could turn it into something decidedly unhappy was terrifying. Could this Trainer #3 experiment be a total gamble, a risk to my love for lifting, or was it exactly what I needed to break through to a whole new level?

By the time I reached the top, my apprehension had given way to cautious optimism. I took a deep breath and started warming up. Ever the professional, Trainer #3 arrived at 6:00 a.m., precisely the time we agreed to meet.

Immediately, I could tell that the intense figure I conjured didn't quite match the man who stood before me. Beneath the intensity was a surprising warmth and an approachability that side-swept my expectations. Yet again, my initial read was completely wrong, and I misjudged him just like I had with Trainer #1 and #2. I pride myself on my ability to read people, a skill honed through years of making staffing decisions. So this consistent inability to accurately size up personal trainers was frustrating and, quite frankly, embarrassing.

Thankfully, I wasn't wrong about Trainer #3's expertise. That was obvious from the first rep. He shared a minor but effective tweak to my form that instantly deepened my connection to the target muscle, allowing me to move more weight with surprising ease. It was a subtle adjustment with a considerable impact.

As we flowed through the workout, the session felt like a masterclass in coaching. Trainer #3 seamlessly blended pinpoint technical cues with perfectly timed encouragement, making me feel challenged and supported.

But despite that huge win, something felt off.

The training itself was all perfectly executed movements and insightful feedback, but the bits between sets were a whole different story. I'm reserved with new people, and when I get too self-conscious, I withdraw even more. What starts as "somewhat unapproachable" quickly lands as "distinctly chilly". Being the perceptive, empathetic guy I now know he is, I'm confident Trainer #3 picked up on my "ice queen" energy. I suspect his professional way of responding was to mirror what he thought was my super-serious, all-business focus with an equal intensity of his own.

The result was a series of awkward moments that are hilarious in hindsight, but in the moment…

Ugh.

This was the best one. Allow me to set the stage.

It's the end of our first session, and I'm trying to look casual while dying on the stair climber. Trainer #3 stood silently on the machine next to me, arms crossed, his face a focused, inscrutable mask. Neither of us spoke. The only sounds were the rhythmic whir of the stair climber and an awful techno remix of "Livin' on a Prayer." The music was the only thing distracting me from the fact that Trainer #3 was studying me with a seriousness that made me feel like I was under a microscope. I'm sure only seconds had ticked by, but each one felt like an eternity as I huffed and puffed up that stairway to nowhere.

My brain immediately filled the silence with a frantic monologue. "Why is he staring at me like that? Is my form that bad? Is it even possible to have bad form on a stair climber? This silence is intense—why can't he just say something? Maybe I should say something. What should I say? Compliment the workout? Too eager. Ask about his workouts? Too nosy. Make a joke about the music? Risky. Okay, Plan B: Bolt for the fire exit the second this machine stops... Where *is* that fire exit again?"

My mind went into overdrive because a part of me recognized that this partnership had the potential to be great. The workout had been challenging and fun, and Trainer #3 was an exceptional coach. I wanted to work with him, so this was an opportunity I couldn't allow to slip through my sweaty fingers.

I *had* to say *something*.

I frantically searched for appropriate topics of conversation. The highest-quality protein powder? The optimal angle for a bicep curl? The existential question of why gyms always play terrible techno remixes of perfectly good 80s songs? At the time, it truly felt to me like a make-it-or-break-it moment straight out of a gym-themed sitcom's season finale cliffhanger.

Will Lisa find the right words and save the day, or will this promising partnership crash and burn in a fiery wreck of social ineptitude?

Maybe it was the tension, the post-workout brain fog, or my low blood sugar after the tough workout he put me through. Whatever the reason, I blurted out the first thing that popped into my oxygen-deprived brain:

"So… Uh… Wanna do this again sometime?"

Smooth, right?

I felt like I was going to vomit. The goal was "cool, confident invitation," but the result was more "icky, desperate, and vaguely inappropriate." My cheeks were on fire. Disappearing into a black hole, never to be seen or heard from again, felt like an appealing option.

How could I ever face him again after that five-star cringe fest?

Against all odds, it didn't send him running. Instead, my epic fail broke the ice. A slow smile spread across his face, and his shoulders visibly relaxed. "How about Thursday?" he replied, his voice laced with just a hint of amusement at my expense.

Over those first few sessions, the initial formality between us softened. We found common ground and connection as we learned more about each other's lives outside the gym. I shared my tales of burnout, divorce drama, blowing up my career, and my lifelong battle with my weight and body image. In turn, Trainer #3 shared stories about the winding path that led him to become the incredible coach and person he is today.

But it was one specific moment of unexpected mutual vulnerability that cleared up the lingering awkwardness between us, and slammed the door shut on my persistent feelings of imposter syndrome for good.

After working together for a few weeks, Trainer #3 and I felt comfortable enough with each other to reminisce about those early awkward moments. That's when we stumbled upon a hilarious truth. He'd seen me training with Trainer #2, day in and day out, lifting weights heavy enough to make a grown man cry. With a sheepish chuckle, he confessed, "I was intimidated by you!"

I nearly did a spit-take with my water. "No way!" I exclaimed, utterly floored. "Are you kidding me? I was intimidated by you, too!" The sheer absurdity of it hit us like a perfectly timed punchline. We both dissolved into laughter, a couple of kindred overthinking spirits, each having hilariously out-worried the other.

Seeing this trainer of champions and the expert who intimidated me as a regular guy wrestling with his own unfounded insecurities, changed how I saw myself. I wasn't fake, phony, or uniquely flawed, and my doubts and fears didn't make me an imposter. They just made me human, part of the flawed majority, like everyone else.

And just like that, laughing with Trainer #3 over how completely wrong we'd been about each other, I felt free to be me, bad jokes, *ridiculous* strength, and all. The whole unfiltered package. From then on, our dynamic shifted, and we settled into the comfortable, easy rhythm of old friends.

Muscle Power, Mind Power Tip #24:
Confessions of a Gym Rat – Why I'll Never
Get Bored of Lifting

I often get asked, with a hint of baffled curiosity, "How do you keep going to the gym, doing the same routines day after day, without getting bored out of your skull?"

I didn't have a great answer beyond the obvious clichés for the longest time. Sure, I loved the feeling of getting stronger, and seeing my body change was fun. But I couldn't quite articulate the deeper reason why my workouts never felt boring or repetitive and always left me feeling energized and excited about the next session.

The answer finally clicked during that first session with Trainer #3. There I was, a confident intermediate lifter with four years of experience under my cute purple suede weightlifting belt, when he blew my mind with a simple tip on my form. It was a tiny technical adjustment but also a humbling reminder that even with all my experience, I still had so much more to learn.

Weight training isn't just about lifting heavy things and putting them back down again until you're tired. It's a skill. A craft, even. I remember one session where Trainer #1 spent ten minutes trying to explain the deadlift. Specifically, that you should push the ground away instead of pulling with your arms. My immediate reaction was a bewildered stare. I was convinced he had officially lost his mind. But with a simple cue and a slight

221

shift in my focus, the lift clicked. The movement felt stronger, more stable, and more powerful than ever before. It's that tiny, almost invisible improvement that keeps me chasing the feeling of mastery.

This mindset works because weight training is endlessly adaptable, meeting you exactly where you are. There's always a clear starting point, a tangible next step, and a new, achievable challenge waiting for you, whether you're a beginner mastering basic movements with soup can weights, or a seasoned athlete tackling complex barbell lifts. There's an incredible, almost addictive satisfaction in nailing a lift that once felt impossible or feeling that perfect mind-muscle connection. This is the *"Mind Power"* secret that keeps my workouts feeling dynamic and engaging, keeping me eagerly coming back for more, year after year.

This principle doesn't just apply to lifting. Whether you're into running, swimming, yoga, dancing, or competitive cheese rolling, adopting a growth mindset can transform your entire experience with movement. When you adopt this mindset, fitness becomes a lifelong practice of continuous learning and growth. The objective isn't to get to a certain number, but to always get a little bit better, stronger, and more capable.

Muscle Power, Mind Power Tip #25:
The Evolution of Goals

Back in November 2019, rocking my trusty Metallica t-shirt and holey jogging pants, I wasn't exactly thrilled with the turn my life had taken. It felt even worse because I didn't love what I saw in the mirror. "If I could just *look* better," I thought, "maybe I'd *feel* better. And if I *felt* better, maybe, just maybe, I could tackle the dumpster fire that is my life."

There's this pervasive and, frankly, misguided bias that chasing health is the only "acceptable" goal, the only "why" deserving of respect. It's like there's a hierarchy of motivation, and aesthetics are stuck at the bottom, labeled as superficial and vain.

But let's be real—how we feel about our appearance impacts how we *feel*, period.

Liking what you see in the mirror boosts confidence, changes how you carry yourself and can be a catalyst for taking better care of yourself overall. We're allowed to care about how we look. Wanting to feel strong, capable, *and* pleased with your reflection is a worthy, multi-faceted goal.

When I first started out, the idea of some future, strong, vital "Grandma Lisa" frolicking with her grandkids felt way too abstract and too far off to grasp, let alone motivate me through a tough workout. But fitting into a pair of jeans that were one size smaller? That felt real, tangible, and something I could wrap my head around now. "Stagnant and Flaccid Lisa" wasn't concerned

223

about things like disease prevention. Her immediate, powerful motivator was simply wanting to feel better about herself by feeling better in her own skin.

But after navigating my health scare and supporting my mom through her cancer treatment and recovery, I came face-to-face with the reality that health isn't a guarantee but a precious gift. That experience was so life-altering that my goals had to shift. That's when "Lifting Lisa" started prioritizing her well-being and healing her relationship with food and exercise.

What motivates us at the starting line might not be what drives us a mile down the road. Clinging to outdated goals that no longer serve the person we are today means we are clinging to an outdated version of ourselves. Our goals should reflect our growth and evolution, guiding us toward a future aligned with our authentic selves and leading us to opportunities we never saw coming.

Sometimes, the most fulfilling paths are the scenic detours we never planned on taking.

I was about to experience that kind of unscripted turn—a third and unexpected shift in my goals. It wasn't something I planned or consciously pursued, at least not at first. It emerged organically, shifting my focus almost without me noticing. I suspect I'll eventually circle back to prioritizing health and longevity, but first, "Lifting Lisa" has some heavy lifting to do!

Trainer #3 (Part 3) – You Are An Athlete (reprised)

Remember when Trainer #2 casually dropped that comment about fueling my body like an athlete?

Back then, fresh off my weight loss journey and still clinging to some old dieting habits, I brushed it off as a motivational tactic, a feel-good compliment that helped me embrace eating healthy, home-cooked meals from plastic containers. While it felt good to be recognized as someone who took their health and fitness seriously, the concept of *being* an athlete felt so far-fetched, so disconnected from my "stagnant and flaccid" history, that the thought didn't even cross my mind.

That changed when I started working with Trainer #3.

He never crossed paths with "Stagnant and Flaccid Lisa," the woman fixated on torching calories for aesthetics. He even missed out on meeting "Lifting Lisa," the woman who discovered a passion for weightlifting and getting *ridiculously* strong, who was motivated by improved health, longevity, and confidence.

The only Lisa he knew was the woman who showed up at the gym day after day, chasing her goals with passion and intensity. From day one, he treated me like I was one of his athletes—a powerlifter with untapped potential.

Trainer #3 wasn't the first to suggest that I compete in powerlifting. In the past, I laughed it off dismissively, perhaps because I wasn't ready to hear it. He even had to bring it up a few times before something finally clicked. But once it did, the idea of stepping onto a platform, testing my limits, and competing against others resonated with my growing confidence and ambition. Even my inner mean girl, who would have normally scoffed at the idea, was strangely quiet.

That's because "Athlete Lisa" was ready to step into the spotlight and rise to the challenge.

So much has changed since my first day in the gym. My perspective on just about everything related to health and fitness has shifted. I've gone from obsessively counting calories to fueling my body with intention, from "restrict and sacrifice" to embracing the basics, from fearing food to seeing it as an ally, from torching calories to training for strength, health, and longevity, from a relentless inner critic to cultivating self-love and acceptance.

I've used the words "journey" and "transformation" a million times throughout this book to describe my life-changing experience. At this point, I can clearly see that they're not only cliché but also wholly inaccurate. Both imply that it will, at some point, come to an end. But I've learned that the "messy middle," the learning and growing part of the process, never ends.

So, what else should I call a complete life overhaul?

A metamorphosis? Too dramatic.

A glow-up? Too Instagram.

It's been more of an epic quest of self-discovery where my inner Katniss Everdeen found her badassery, met up with Brené Brown for a deep dive into vulnerability, then grabbed a pint with Bridget Jones to master self-deprecating humor and self-acceptance, all while channeling Elle Woods to defy every expectation.

If I knew then what I know now, I might have used "evolution," because it implies an ongoing process and a continuous unfolding of potential. And that's precisely what this experience has been for me.

My point is that I'm not some finished product, neatly packaged and tied with a bow. I'm still learning, growing, and figuring things out as I go. And that's the beauty of it. There is no finish line, just a constant state of *becoming*. It's in those uncertain spaces, between who we are and who we're striving to be, that we truly discover ourselves, push our boundaries, and uncover strengths we never knew we had.

And honestly? I couldn't be more excited for what's next.

Will I become a powerlifting champion, gracing your social media feed with my bulging biceps and inspirational quotes about lifting heavy things?

Anything is possible!

The one thing I know for sure is that the next step in my evolution will be filled with valuable lessons, delightfully unexpected detours, and moments of pure joy.

Though this adventure began with a blind pursuit of weight loss at any cost, it evolved into a quest to become the best version of myself, inside and out. It became about embracing every messy, imperfect step along the way—the endless possibilities, the unknown paths stretching out before me, and the chance to surprise myself over and over again.

The "messy middle" is where I live now. It's where I thrive and where I continue to evolve. It's a place of learning, growth, and self-discovery where I'm constantly redefining my limits and rewriting my story.

I hope you'll join me there.

Let's embrace the unique, imperfect, and endlessly fascinating experience of becoming our best selves, together.

Acknowledgements

To my reader: Sharing my story has been an exercise in vulnerability, so I'm so grateful that you stuck with me through every sweaty workout, car-crying session, and run-in with my inner mean girl. You're more than just a reader; you're a confidante who held space for my story and a fellow traveler on this messy path of *becoming*. I hope my stumbles and successes help you on your way. I'll be cheering you on, always.

To the amazing staff at my gym, who have become my friends: You might not realize the impact of your daily kindness, but in an environment that can feel intimidating, your genuine smiles and easy "good mornings" (the greeting, not the hamstring killer!) always made walking through the door feel welcoming. Thank you for the countless times you stopped by my corner table in the lobby to share a moment while I spent hours writing there. You transformed the gym lobby into a space that felt as comfortable and familiar as my living room. It was a crucial "third place" where I felt safe and supported while tackling this project. That sense of community is something I'll never forget.

To Trainer #3: Thank you for being the only person I felt comfortable sharing an early version of this messy manuscript with. It's a level of trust I wouldn't have predicted on our day one, as I mentally located the nearest fire exit! Beyond the killer programming and technique tweaks, you held me accountable to my training *and* this deeply personal dream I've carried for most of my life. You knew when to ask the tough questions that kept me moving forward when I wanted to stall. That support means more than you know.

To my friends and family: Where would I be without you? Thank you for asking thoughtful questions about the book (even when you were probably sick of hearing about it!), listening without judgment as I rambled through half-formed ideas, and being my essential sounding board and constant source of inspiration. Knowing I had you in my corner helped me shape this book into something I'm deeply proud to share. I couldn't have done it without your love and encouragement.

About the Author

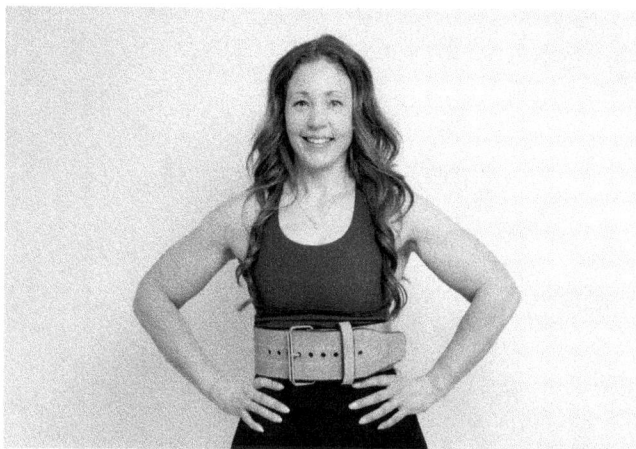

Living in Ottawa, Ontario, with her partner Serge, his two boys, Patrick and Justin, Justin's girlfriend Naomie, and their adorable Morkie, Bailey, Lisa's life is never dull. Her blended family is a whirlwind of fun, love, and the everyday adventures that keep things interesting. Her journey through weight loss opened her eyes to the world of weight training. Now, she focuses on embracing her inner badass, and helping others through the messy process of *becoming* by sharing what she learned.

www.ingramcontent.com/pod-product-compliance
Lightning Source LLC
Chambersburg PA
CBHW051717020426
42333CB00014B/1021